"Dr. Joyce Starr reveals the **rejùvenating and life-sustaining power of healthy salt**. This creative work should be embraced by health-seekers and salt lovers worldwide."

– Black Tai Salt Company
www.BlackTaiSaltCo.com

"**Dr. Joyce Starr's book delivers! You won't want to place this book on the shelf and leave it there!** Her knowledge of salt for healing is at your finger tips. **I highly recommend this book to help you create the best possible solution** for healing and clearing any space in your home or offices."

– Yvonne Phillips, FSII
www.FengShuiPublications.com

"This work serves up a wonderful buffet of **salt facts and salt enlightenment**. I can't wait to indulge in the healing salt therapies included in the book."

– Nicole Onley, Maryland

"*Salt Secrets* **heralds the pristine beauty within.** The energy of life is revealed in glorious detail, while the **wisdom is priceless.**"

– Victor H. Rodriguez, Washington, D.C.

"Thank you so much for the information on how to make the Salt Solution from natural salt crystals. **I look forward to a healthier body and life.** You've been such a gift in your sharing."

– Karen A., California

"Your sensational work is **now required reading** for my entire family."

– C. Powers, Maryland

"This invaluable work helps me spread the word to family, friends and clients."

– Lilly Neff, Arizona

Salt Secrets

Salt Tips For Life

Dr. Joyce Starr

Salt is Born of the Purest of Parents:
the Sun and the Sea.

– Pythagoras

Salt Secrets
Salt Tips for Life

Dr. Joyce Starr

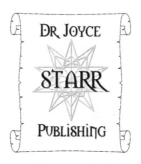

www.DrJoyceStarr.com

Publisher: Dr. Joyce STARR Publishing
www.DrJoyceStarr.com
Aventura, Florida
Phone: 1-786-693-4223

Published in the United States of America.

© 2006 by Dr. Joyce Starr. All Rights Reserved.

No part of this book may be used or reproduced, stored in a retrieval system, or transmitted in any form or by any means, electronic, mechanical, photocopying, recording or otherwise, except in the case of brief quotations embodied in articles or reviews and as permitted under Section 107 or 108 of the 1976 United States Copyright Act, without the prior permission of the publisher.

ISBN 10 - 0-9792333-1-3
ISBN 13 - 978-0-9792333-1-9

This book is available for special promotions. Contact: info@drjoycestarr.com

First Edition – 2007

Cover Design by Be Mused Author Services
www.BeMusedAuthor.com

DISCLAIMER

While the publisher and author have used their best efforts in preparing this book, they make no representation or warranties with respect to the accuracy or completeness of the contents of this book and specifically disclaim any implied warranties of merchantability or fitness for a particular purpose. No warranty may be created or extended by sales representatives or written sales materials. The advice and strategies contained herein may not be suitable for your situation. The publisher is not engaged in rendering professional services, and you should consult with a professional where appropriate. Neither the publisher nor the author shall be liable for any loss of profit or any other commercial damages, including but not limited to special, incidental, consequential or other damages.

Dr. Starr is not a medical practitioner and does not dispense medical advice. This work is based on public documents and on her personal experiences. The views expressed by the author are solely her opinion.

SPECIAL APPRECIATION

To my mother, for the gift of determination and steady belief in the improbable, and to my father, for the treasure of his wit and the unswerving conviction that tomorrow will be a better day.

To Dave Goldenberg, for generous review of numerous drafts.

To Jonathan D, for creative and scientific contributions – and for images that have taken on a life of their own.

To Wynette A. Hoffman, for invaluable publishing insights and for a cover design so inviting that I want to sail away to the Natural Salt Oasis.

The Crystal

Then the miracle, that molten sand melts
Into the most beautiful crystalline
Form, a transparent jewel, a marvel,
Liquefied jade, gossamer amethyst
Ruby, Emerald, Jasper, Mother of Pearl.
Radiant colors, tissue thin material,
Both of light and form. Like the bulb
Around a light, it shines, but now
Warm, its ghostly form dissolves to
Reveal an inmost beating heart.
Wraith, no longer, but the marrow
Of love, the spirit of life, the soul.
Of your soul.

– Dr. Prem Deben

DEDICATION

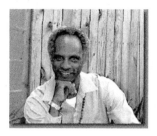

This work is dedicated to my beloved friend and spiritual guide, Dr. Prem Deben ('Deben'), who departed his body in 2006 at the peak of his journey – far too early for those who felt safest when he embraced their world.

Deben introduced me to the wide panorama of self-healing possibilities. He scoured the planet for ancient healing wisdom that could help illuminate the path of those who arrived at his door.

He was also a story-teller. Deben wrote: "I live to tell stories that will bring about deep transformations in the lives of people I'm honored to serve." Healer, scientist, poet, scholar and guru. Advanced healing technologies, the Bible or the fruits of life – he was a master of all.

Ever generous with empathy and insight, he gently but persistently challenged all seekers to wrestle with the twin question: Who are you, and how do you plan to live your journey?

He left many devotees speechless – one mourner after another expressing the frustration that mortal words could not capture how much their lives had been transformed by his wisdom, by his healing and by his heart.

On one occasion, he left an audio tape at the desk of my building. The tape contained an ethereal soundtrack with a single refrain: "Return to the land of your soul."

I pray that you are in high spirits, dearest Deben, in the land of your soul.

CONTENTS

Section I: The Natural Salt Oasis

Section II: Salt Tips for Life

PREFACE

My first e-Book on natural salt healing – *Himalayan Salt Crystals: Your Dynamic Wellness Guide* – was warmly received. Plans for a paperback version were in progress. But something held me back.

Wellness issues are so often couched in pseudo-scientific jargon that the myriad of claims and promises are nearly impossible to comprehend, let alone validate. I wanted to take a fresher, more imaginative approach that beginners and practitioners alike could easily absorb.

Daydreaming in my kitchen one morning, I heard the faint whisper of Deben's Tennessee lilt. "The voice of salt," he said. "Why not invite the original natural salt guru to help convey your message?"

Had Deben cooked up a new recipe for my readers? What better site than the kitchen to transmit the perfect salt solution: a blend of ancient salt wisdom sweetened with practical salt tips for body, spirit and home. I hope you enjoy the rather unusual formula for salt wealth health.

For you and your descendants, this is a Covenant of Salt forever before God.

– Book of Numbers 18:19

Salt Secrets: Salt Tips for Life

INTRODUCTION

Nay: "There is no introduction."

Say: "How can you introduce a story without an introduction?"

Nay: "I explained that to you once before."

Say: "Can you tell me again?"

Nay: "Humans are in a hurry; they don't have time for introductions. Now please be quiet. Not another word."

Say: "Can I sing?"

Nay: "No distractions."

Say: "But I want to help."

Nay: "Then help me lower the curtain before it's too late."

Say: "But I thought the story begins late."

Salt Secrets: Salt Tips for Life

Nay: "Yes, but not too late."

Say: "So it's best to start early when you want to be late?"

Nay: "The bedroom drape is closing. Now don't speak, don't sing and please don't ask another irrelevant question."

Say: "What if I have an answer?"

Salt Secrets: Salt Tips for Life

✳ One ✳

YOUR SALT GURU

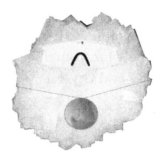

"Let me introduce myself. NaCl is my given name. I'm also known as the King's Salt, table salt and simply salt, but my closest friends call me Nacell. I was given birth over a quarter of a billion years ago by the Primal Sea of Planet Earth – which makes me the child of the source of life.

"I have an especially rich history. As the Roman statesman Cassiodorus observed, 'Some seek not gold, but there lives not a man who does not need salt.' Indeed, I was once more valuable than gold.

Salt Secrets: Salt Tips for Life

"In ancient China, I was in such high demand that they molded me into coins. In fact, as you can see, I'm wearing the first ancient salt coin ever produced. When impersonators vie for my place in history, I simply take it with a grain of salt.

"But enough about me. To help you understand the meaning of salt for your life, I must first tell you about Jasmine and Crystal.

"Jasmine is a single woman with a wealthy name. Indeed, according to Renaissance legend, a flowering Jasmine plant is a harbinger of prosperity. Unfortunately, Jasmine has yet to achieve that promise. Both her health and bank account are declining by the day.

"An aspiring graphic artist, Jasmine was hired by a top advertising firm straight out of college, earning a handsome income after a handful of years. A decade later, mercurial bosses, cutthroat co-workers and unforgiving clients had her spirit in an every-tightening vise.

"At the age of 37, she made a bold decision to start a home based business and work only for clients

Salt Secrets: Salt Tips for Life

that she liked. Fast forward five years. Jasmine is glued to her computer nearly fourteen hours a day – working so hard that she doesn't even have time to miss the life she's missing. Her neck and back ache constantly, while bolts of pain run down her legs at night from endless sitting. She takes a walk every evening, but it's not enough.

"Jasmine worries that she has lost the physical ability to rebound from flat out fatigue to high gear on demand. If she's this exhausted now, how will she feel next year and the year thereafter?

"Her best client – the only one that pays invoices on time – hawks pain killers for incurable diseases. Nice people, but the work makes her sick. Dreams of creative work that she adores all but evaporated over the past few years. Lack of money is now a draining fixation.

"As for Jasmine's social life, Mr. Right turned left eons ago, while most of her friends are burping babies and diapering the remains of earnest careers. She often awakes in tears and has never felt so alone in her life.

Salt Secrets: Salt Tips for Life

"Crystal is her closest companion. A ball of long white fur with keen orange eyes, the cat doesn't walk, she bounces – frequently leaping into the air from a standing position for no discernable reason.

"Pet-mom and cat are both keenly attuned to the sound of beating hearts. In the micro-second that Jasmine's spirit awakens to the new day, Crystal leaps onto her pillow to mew a morning greeting. Jasmine often stops what she's doing in the middle of the day just to absorb the gentle percussion of Crystal's sleepy breathing. They're a good team.

"Crystal, however, is more than meets the eye. Indeed, this white bundle of energy is actually a salt angel in disguise, with the power to transport her beloved pet-mom to the oasis of internal wealth. A worthy goal, but for one major obstacle: Crystal is not permitted to move an inch until Jasmine asks the universe for help.

"Poor Crystal has been waiting patiently for seven years, six months, five days, four hours and three minutes – but who is counting? Yet, to Crystal's frustration, Jasmine rarely asks the universe for assistance, and when she does, it's for practical matters: 'Help me find my keys.' 'Where are my glasses?' Could it get any more boring?

"But here's the wonderful news: Jasmine's journey is about to begin at any moment. I have it on high authority that she will ask for intervention this very evening! And in that mystical moment – the rich space between what was and what can be – she will be transported to our **Natural Salt Oasis**, a parallel dimension visible only to those with a deep desire for transformation.

"You can't imagine the fuss. We receive so few visitors that when a new wellness seeker arrives, our little community virtually explodes with connectivity. Naturally, I'm ecstatic. I can't wait to show off my higher frequency."

"Dear reader, you are the only one – absolutely the only one – I can tell about Jasmine's salt journey. Can you keep a secret?"

Salt Secrets: Salt Tips for Life

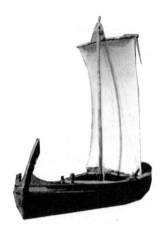

✯ Two ✯

YOUR SALT OASIS

Hugging her pillow for a deeper level of sleep, Jasmine fell out of bed and hit the floor with a thud.

Shocked into consciousness, she made a quick mental check for bruises. All body parts seemed to be intact. The room slowly came into focus. Where was her bed? Where was her bedroom? Jasmine was flat on her back on the cold floor of what appeared to be an ancient wooden sail boat.

She blinked several times. A jagged white crystal sporting designer sunglasses and a gold coin around its neck treaded water to the right of the craft. "Ahoy there," exclaimed Nacell. He spent days practicing the perfect greeting and tone.

The crystalline figure seemed to steer the boat from his position in the water. Even more absurd,

Salt Secrets: Salt Tips for Life

Jasmine was certain that it spoke to her. "Where am I?" she dared to ask.

Nacell was overjoyed. It had been far too long since he engaged in human conversation! "You're on the Primal Sea, the sea of life," he proudly declared. "The Primal Sea nurtured the first living cell and all subsequent life on this planet. Those fortunate enough to discover its wealth are wealthy indeed."

White puffs of salt danced on blue-green waters as far as the eye could see. "Why am I here?" Jasmine persisted.

"You're here," explained Nacell, "because you finally asked the universe for help. Surely you remember? You prayed last night that your physical pains would vanish, you would regain your energy and that you would be overwhelmed by riches. What a relief! After all those years of unnecessary stress and struggle, you finally began your true journey. Of course, Crystal had something to do with it..."

Salt Secrets: Salt Tips for Life

"What have you done to my cat?" Jasmine looked around for something she could use to defend herself.

"Crystal is a higher nature spirit," said Nacell in a soft, reassuring voice. "When you asked for help, she instantly transported you to our Natural Salt Oasis. We don't receive many visitors. You will be treated to a gold carpet."

"You mean a red carpet?"

"We don't have red carpets here. They're all made of gold. Salt was once so valuable that we obtained an ounce of gold for an ounce of salt. Since we controlled the market on salt, we naturally traded salt for gold. Today, salt is relatively inexpensive, but in certain circumstances – for example, if you don't have the proper salt balance in your body – all the gold in the world will not replace your salt. And Crystal is fine. She's waiting for you at our first stop: It's almost here!"

"In other words, we're almost there?"

Salt Secrets: Salt Tips for Life

"No, yes, not quite – it's almost here, but you're not yet there."

Enraged by this doublespeak, Jasmine made a quick assessment. She was stranded in a wooden boat on the so-called sea of life, speaking to a jagged salt crystal with impeccable English. She clearly bruised her head when she fell out of bed.

"I sense your confusion," Nacell interjected, aware that humans calm down when others identify with their emotions. "You can't reach the Natural Salt Oasis on your own. It only appears when you're ready to enter."

"And who are you?" Jasmine demanded.

"Please forgive me. I was so elated to welcome a human guest that I completely forgot my manners. My given name is NaCl. I'm also known as Halite, salt, table salt or by my chemical name in consumable form. In ancient times, they called me the King of Salt.

"The truth is that I'm a combination of the two elements, sodium and chlorine. When these two

Salt Secrets: Salt Tips for Life

elements combine by sharing electrons to form a molecule of Halite, chemists call me sodium chloride. My chloride side is about 10 percent heavier. I hope the extra weight doesn't show," he coyly added. "But I prefer that you call me Nacell after my chemical formula, which is based on the atomic symbols for my elements: Na for sodium and Cl for chlorine.

"The words sodium and chlorine date back to the time when chemists named elements in Greek and Latin. Chlorine derives from the Greek term 'chloros' or greenish yellow. Sodium also derives from the Greek word 'natrium' or soda. Whatever you do, please do not call me chloros natrium. It's simply Greek to me.

"What matters most is that I'm essential to all life on earth. A human body can't manufacture sodium, yet your body requires sodium to transport nutrients, oxygen and nerve impulses.

"I couldn't care less about salt." Jasmine blinked back tears of frustration. "I demand that you take me home.

Salt Secrets: Salt Tips for Life

"Your world is salt, and your home is an oasis," Nacell continued. "But here's the problem: You can't leave until you arrive. You can't arrive until you see, and you can't see until you ask the right question.

"And please do not think about rocking the boat or jumping ship until you reach firmer ground. If you fall overboard, I'll be compelled to dive in and rescue you. Then we'll both be neck-deep in primal stew."

Nacell glistened with pride at the pun.

✫ Three ✫

YOUR SALT CONVEYOR

"**W**hat question?" Jasmine persisted, determined to keep him focused. "And what can I possibly learn at the Natural Salt Oasis?"

"That's precisely the right question! A desert oasis provides nourishment in the wilderness," Nacell explained, "while the Natural Salt Oasis offers nourishing respite from the wilderness of self-defeating habits."

"What's wrong with my habits?"

Nacell wasn't about to let her change the subject. He'd worked on this script for weeks. Raising his voice several octaves, he proclaimed: "The Primal Sea contained all the water that existed on this planet prior to life. Was that sea salty? Yes! At one point this planet was covered by a boiling body of salty water.

Salt Secrets: Salt Tips for Life

"As the water cooled down and a shift to arctic conditions caused glaciers to form, the oceans receded, leaving salt beds behind. Randomly scattered particles of salt slowly drifted towards the bottom of the water, forming crystalline structures or what scientists call a tightly bound molecules.

"In a dry state, these molecules appear as crystals of various sizes, shapes and colors. A diamond, for example, is tightly formed carbon. Glass is tightly formed silicon. Sodium and chlorine, the two building blocks of salt, combine to form a tightly bound molecule. Baby salt crystals are nearly perfect cubes. As the salt crystal matures and attracts other salt crystals, it takes on different forms. Look at me: I'm no longer square!"

Jasmine was stone-faced. Nacell looked frantically for a sea mineral that could give him a quick burst of adrenalin. "Salt crystals are typically joined together in a matrix. They stack left, right and on top of one another. A single salt molecule that can tread water alone in the ocean is quite a rare phenomenon," he said proudly.

Salt Secrets: Salt Tips for Life

Peering over the edge, Jasmine discovered that the boat was resting atop an expansive salt dune. They were no longer moving.

"Your Natural Salt Oasis is approaching," said Nacell, "Please step out of the boat and onto the Salt Conveyor. We can't waste time."

"But I don't see anything. Where are we going?"

"You can walk alongside if you prefer, but please try and keep up with me. I must convey information as fast as possible."

"How can I be sure that you will bring me back to where we are now?" Jasmine asked.

"Indeed, you're right," said Nacell. "Hopefully, you'll be so transformed by your journey that you won't want to return to where you began."

"I'm referring to the boat," she said through pinched lips, "When can I go home?"

Salt Secrets: Salt Tips for Life

"Soon enough," declared Nacell. "But since you haven't stepped out of the boat you're in, how can you go back before you go forward?"

Grimacing, Jasmine placed one leg over the side of the craft. "Wonderful, wonderful," Nacell cheered. "What do you think of our Salt Brick Conveyor?"

Jasmine was taken aback by the stunning mix of red, yellow, pink and white hues. "Are these actual salt bricks?"

"You're standing on authentic salt crystal remnants of the Primal Sea," he proudly declared. "We call it Mother Nature's art."

"But this salt is so colorful? I thought that all salt was white."

"It depends on the presence of inclusions in the particular environment where the salt crystals are formed," Nacell explained. "Have you ever noticed a tiny inclusion in a diamond or a minute piece of garnet caught in the carbon matrix of a gemstone? Inclusions – often referred to as impurities – determine color. Inclusions distinguish a ruby

Salt Secrets: Salt Tips for Life

from a sapphire, or an emerald from an aquamarine. All gems are rocks, including salt crystals. You might say that salt really rocks!" Jasmine tried hard not to laugh.

"My natural color is clear or cloudy white, but I can also assume a variety of colors, including pink, red, orange, yellow, brown, black or even blue. The color of salt depends on inclusions found in the original deposits."

"The salt conveyor bricks appear to be identical in shape." Jasmine remarked. "You can't possibly expect me to believe that they're natural."

"You caught me on that one!"Nacell smiled. "Let me explain. Salt deposits typically derive from salt found in seas, oceans and salt lakes. Therefore, you can still find Primal Sea remnants in salt deposits around the world, including those ancient caves where sedimentary salt evaporated eons ago.

"Our Salt Brick Conveyor, for example, is actually made up of thousands of salt rocks drawn from salt caves located over 500 feet beneath the

Salt Secrets: Salt Tips for Life

Himalayan Mountain Range, from salt caves in Poland and from salt caves in other parts of the world.

"These ancient salt blocks were mined by hand, rather than with explosives. Craftsmen then transformed the salt blocks into a variety of wonderful shapes, including salt crystal lamps, salt crystal candleholders and even decorative salt tiles for walls and floors.

"Now here's the important point: Inclusions in the salt environment can be both positive and negative for your health. If the inclusions are poisonous, the salt will be poisonous as well, irrespective of where it was discovered. When it comes to salt that you ingest, the question is: Does the salt contain inclusions, and if so, are these inclusions positive for your health? Are they both edible and eatable? Edible substances provide nutritional value, while eatable materials pass through your system without doing harm.

"The Japanese frequently garnish their food with gold leaf to give it a lustrous appearance. Martha Stewart enjoys painting cakes and cookies with specks of gold. Gold is eatable, but not digestible and therefore not edible. A heavy metal that is not used by the body, gold has absolutely no nutritional value. Eating gold could deplete your wealth and will not improve your health. Salt, by contrast, is priceless. You must ingest salt to survive."

Nacell congratulated himself on delivering the perfect sound-bite. Jasmine was still agitating over the Salt Brick Conveyor. "Bricks cannot possibly float on the sea's surface," she insisted, "much less move forward like a conveyor belt. What if the conveyor collapses? We'll drown!"

Salt Secrets: Salt Tips for Life

There's nobody left but God....
Maybe He knows the cure:
Not a mouthful my little one takes.
Ah, he will die for sure.

There is no salt in the house,
Never a pinch of it here.
"Try some flour," said God.
God whispered it in my ear.

The little one took a bite,
He made a face as he bit.
He cried, the tiny boy:
"Put more salt on it!"

I floured the crust again,
My tears rained on the bread.
The little one ate it up,
The little son was fed.

She boasted of her ruse:
She had saved him, it appears.
Ah, mother, mother,
Those were salty tears!

– Ivan Turgenev

✵ Four ✵

YOUR SALT CONDUCTOR

"**S**alt is the conductor of your destiny and the ancient treasures within." Nacell responded. "You can leave the ocean, but it will never leave you. Man, fish, reptiles, birds and mammals carry sodium, potassium, and calcium within their blood in almost the same proportion as the oceans.

"Even fresh-water fish contain almost the identical salt balance found in the sea. In fact, to keep fresh-water fish healthy, you must add one tablespoon of salt per five gallons of aquarium water. Fish, like humans, are natural salt eaters."

"Where do fresh-water fish obtain their salt?" Jasmine puzzled.

"From rainfall and rocks. Rain dissolves salt deposits hidden in rocks," he explained. Water is vital to life, yet you can still survive for three days without ingesting water. By contrast, you cannot

Salt Secrets: Salt Tips for Life

survive for a second without salt in your body. Salt helps regulate, maintain and balance the exchange of water between your cells and their surrounding fluids. The correct salinity rate in your body – your internal level of salt conductivity – makes it possible for your cells to work effectively.

"Salt assists in the formation and proper functioning of the nerve fibers that send impulses to and from you brain. Salt also helps you digest food and helps your heart beat correctly. Salt is your natural internal pacemaker.

"Your metabolism is regulated by sodium, calcium, magnesium and potassium. Salt combines with potassium to regulate the acid-alkaline balance in your blood. Salt also helps your muscles work at peak efficiency. The sodium component of salt (Na) is involved in muscle contractions, including your heartbeat, nerve impulses and the digestion of proteins. Your muscular system will not function without salt, or to be accurate, without approximately 50 percent of salt."

Salt Secrets: Salt Tips for Life

"Fifty percent?" Jasmine repeated. Now she was totally confused."

"Salt is comprised of both Na (sodium) and Cl (chlorine). Therefore, it stands to reason that only 50 percent of your salt might be needed at any given time."

"Humans and animals alike experience different symptoms from having too much salt or not having enough salt – both are equally bad. If you don't have enough salt in your body, you feel exhausted, dizzy and your muscles ache. Fortunately, your body automatically stores a bit of salt each day," he added.

"Most people love salt so much – indeed they so addicted to salt – that too little salt is typically not a problem. But you also lose salt every day. Therefore, if you remain on absolutely salt free diet and ingest food that has no salt content whatsoever, you will slowly die. Just as humans can perish from too little water, they can also perish from too little salt, though your internal salt drought may not be felt as quickly."

Salt Secrets: Salt Tips for Life

"How can I tell if I have the right amount of salt?" Jasmine asked.

"If you have too little salt, your salt balance declines along with your health. Ingest too much salt and your body dissipates the excess. If you ingest more salt than your body can dissipate, your salt level starts to rise – resulting in a myriad of health problems. For example, the Great Salt Lake in Utah and Israel's Dead Sea contain so much salt that it eventually killed the fish, the plants and finally the sea. Are you thirsty?" Nacell inquired.

"I'm absolutely parched!"

Nacell handed her a cup full of white powder. "But this is salt," she grimaced.

"No, it's your salt," Nacell responded. "The salt in this cup represents the amount of salt in your body – between four and eight ounces at any given time, depending on a variety of factors." He quickly produced a cup of water. "If you fail to drink water and consume too much salt, the salt could harm you."

Salt Secrets: Salt Tips for Life

He poured a good bit of salt into the cup of water. "Salt floats in water, but the crystals are so small that you can't see them moving. In fact, if you hold seawater up to the light, it seems a bit cloudy. The clouds are minute salts, baby salts – little bitty salt. Liquid – in this case water – allows the surface of salt to dissolve, and it is now free to move or to float in the water.

"You might say that salt treads water, although in general there is usually more salt at the bottom of a glass. In any case you should never ingest more then a teaspoon of salt a day. I guess you've heard of bipolar personalities. Well, salt is also bipolar – meaning that one side is different than the other. A magnet has both a north and a south pole. A molecular unit of salt has a positive and negative side. You might think of salt poles like a twisted balloon, with one side larger than the other.

"Salt conducts electricity in your body by allowing other electrons to dance on its surface. In turn, these electrons make it possible for your internal electricity to pass from point A to point B."

Salt Secrets: Salt Tips for Life

Nacell tried to squeeze his sunglasses up a notch. "Which mineral inclusions do you want in your cup of salt? Which mineral inclusions does your body need or crave?

"For example, do you want ancient sea salt inclusions, table salt inclusions or kosher salt inclusions? If your food or vitamins contain large amounts of magnesium, and your salt includes a great deal of magnesium as well, you could unintentionally ingest too much magnesium through your salt."

Jasmine frowned. "I use those little packets of salt offered with fast food take outs. What type of salt is that? "

Nacell launched into his Salt 101 monologue. "There are basically two kinds of salt: sea salt and rock salt. Sea salt is evaporated and distilled from seawater, while rock salt is typically found in salt rock deposits. Rock salt is usually – though not always – gray in color with many beneficial impurities.

Salt Secrets: Salt Tips for Life

"Table salt is refined rock salt, while Kosher salt is refined rock salt with lime inclusions. Salt sold in supermarkets or that comes in packets is often processed to the point that it contains very little aside from salt," he said. "Various salt brands contain additives and preservatives to prevent caking or sugar to improve the flavor.

"Moreover, 70 percent of all table salt includes minuscule amounts of iodine to prevent hypothyroidism or goiters – also known as an enlarged thyroid. Iodine was added to American table salt in the 1920s when hypothyroidism was nearly at epidemic levels and removed when consumers complained about the inclusion. Hypothyroidism is almost nonexistent today, while iodine deficiency is on the rise in the United States.

"There are differing rules around the world about just which inclusions and how many edible inclusions salt can have – and also what names you can use for salt. You can often distinguish one edible salt from another by the size of its grain structure and by its inclusions."

Salt Secrets: Salt Tips for Life

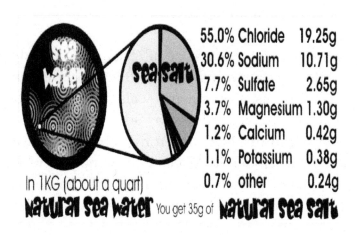

55.0%	Chloride	19.25g
30.6%	Sodium	10.71g
7.7%	Sulfate	2.65g
3.7%	Magnesium	1.30g
1.2%	Calcium	0.42g
1.1%	Potassium	0.38g
0.7%	other	0.24g

In 1KG (about a quart) **Natural sea water** You get 35g of **Natural sea salt**

✵ Five ✵

YOUR SALT HUNGER

Jasmine was growing weary. "Do I really need to know all of this?"

"Do you hunger for purple or green salt?" Nacell responded.

"Purple salt is produced when a particular French flower gives off pollen, the pollen rests on the surface of salt beds and is actually trapped in the salt matrix while it forms.

"When you place salt in water, it begins as a suspension. A limited amount of water can only hold so much salt before it reaches saturation. If you pour saturated water into a pan, it's rich in salt.

As the water evaporates, crystallized salt coats the bottom of the pan. If you put healthy greens or even green food color into the salt water, the green

Salt Secrets: Salt Tips for Life

color is caught in the salt matrix. And thus you have green salt. White or clear salt from the Dead, by contrast, carries inclusions that do not affect the color.

"While there are numerous salt facts you can happily choose to ignore, others could enhance the quality your life – salt as culinary art, for example. A dish often tastes best at a five-star restaurant because the chef employs the best artisan salt. Leading restaurants offer sorbet or wine to clear the palate between entrees. Some also provide a treasure cove of artisan salt dips between courses.

"I had no idea that food salt could be so interesting," Jasmine declared.

Nacell persevered. "Various salt crystal shapes present more or less salt to the tongue. The more salt that contacts your tongue, the more salt you taste. Even if you lick the surface of a large salt cube, you will likely taste less than one billionth of the salt.

"Doctors warn that salt contributes to high blood pressure, but there is no proof that excess salt in a

Salt Secrets: Salt Tips for Life

healthy person causes direct harm. Conversely, no one has proven that excess salt will do you any good. People who suffer from inner ear disorders or vertigo – acute sea or motion sickness and dizziness while standing still on dry land – should definitely avoid excess salt.

"Your kidneys regulate the percentage of salt in your body and thus in most cases protect you from excess salt. By the same token, your kidneys also work overtime to remove that excess – irrespective of the type of salt you ingest. Even the healthiest salt is unhealthy if consumed in excess of what your body can process or what it needs.

"I haven't been feeling so well lately," Jasmine admitted. "I'm exhausted and stressed out most of the time."

"Your body could be suffering from too much salt, too little salt or from a lack of minerals that your salt does not provide," said Nacell. "We've established that you must have salt to live, that sodium is an essential mineral and that salt can also contain other vital mineral inclusions.

Salt Secrets: Salt Tips for Life

"So the question is, what other minerals does your body need to operate at peak efficiency? Can you obtain and can your body actually process those minerals from the food or vitamins that you ingest? Not all vitamins are easily digestible. You might require additional minerals just to process the supplement. Therefore, the salt that is best for you depends on the salt you need."

"Which inclusions I need? I have no time for this." She was once again frustrated and annoyed.

"You can take various medical tests to determine which minerals you lack or try a simple home experiment," Nacell counseled. "Use a particular salt for a few weeks. If you feeling better, there's a good chance that the salt contains mineral inclusions that your body craves. Just be certain that you don't ingest an excessive amount of salt in the process. People often purchase expensive 'designer' salt for home use and then absorb unlimited amounts of salt from fast food lunches or store-bought meals. The trick is to take control, to understand how much salt you ingest daily and then to decide how much salt you really need. It's a fine balance.

Salt Secrets: Salt Tips for Life

"But there's another solution," Nacell loved double entendres. "You can also create a natural salt drink packed with minerals."

"Drink salt?"

"Yes, that's right," said Nacell. "You can mix up a potent natural Salt Solution by dissolving several mineral rich Himalayan salt crystal rocks in pure water and let the rocks dissolve for twenty-four hours. Water absorbs the mineral inclusions in the salt crystal.

"The water is 'salt saturated' when the rocks no longer dissolve. You can then mix a teaspoon of the salty brine water in eights ounces of quality mineral water for an energy-packed drink."

Jasmine was intrigued. "Is the salt in our body a mineral, a chemical or an element? And does it really matter whether we use one salt or another to take a bath?"

"Excellent questions!" Nacell was energized by her sudden interest. "Salt is always a mineral, including the salt in your body. Indeed, you might

Salt Secrets: Salt Tips for Life

think of salt as a high-class mineral that aids digestion by increasing the hydrochloric acid content of digestive fluids.

"Salt crystals can also contain elements, minerals or even chemicals," he continued. "An element is an atom or atomic structure – and every atom is an element of the periodic table. But not all elements provide nutritional value. A grain of sand might contain thousands of elemental silicone atoms, but you wouldn't want to dine on a meal of sand.

"And yes, the salt you choose for bathing does matter. Epsom Salt, Dead Sea salt and Himalayan salt are all especially relaxing and revitalizing when used for bathing.

"Humans discovered the healing properties of Epsom Salt about a century ago and have been using them ever since to help relax sore muscles. Make no mistake. Epsom salts and table salts are not one and the same. Epsom salts contain magnesium, while table salt does not.

"The body welcomes certain elements. Magnesium is a welcomed visitor – even a life saving visitor –

Salt Secrets: Salt Tips for Life

if you have a magnesium deficiency. It can be absorbed directly through the skin. Magnesium plays an important role in transporting calcium deposits out of the body. The body also needs magnesium to bind adequate amounts of serotonin, a mood-elevating brain chemical that creates a feeling of calm and relaxation. Magnesium also acts as a diacritic if ingested, but should not be ingested without medical supervision.

"The salt-concentrated waters of the Dead Sea have provided curative relief for sufferers of psoriasis and other skin ailments for thousands of years, while a float in the Dead Sea is guaranteed to reduce mental and physical stress.

"Himalayan salt was discovered in salt caves deep beneath the Himalayan Mountain Range in ancient times and is now a popular healing remedy in Asia, Europe and the United States. Some report dramatic improvements in soft tissue ailments if they drink the salt brine solution on a regular basis and wrap sore muscles in a wet towel saturated with Himalayan salt. Relaxing in a lukewarm Himalayan salt bath is energizing and

Salt Secrets: Salt Tips for Life

rejuvenating for skin, body and spirit. Indeed, a regular bathing regime of Dead Sea Salt, Epsom Salt and Himalayan Salt can be quite beneficial. But don't combine them in one bath solution!

"Numerous face and body creams, soaps and masks also contain Dead Sea salt, Himalayan salt and a variety of healing salts from around the world. The therapeutic benefits of one salt versus another largely depend on the mineral inclusions (or lack thereof) in that salt – combined with your body's hunger for those particular inclusions at a given time."

Nacell took a deep breath. His silence didn't last very long.

✯ Six ✯

YOUR SALT FREQUENCY

"**B**alance is everything," Nacell continued. "Just as our boat must be balanced to keep you afloat, your internal salt must be balanced to keep you healthy."

Jasmine realized that the conveyor hadn't moved an inch. She was still standing next to the boat. "The conveyor is broken."

"To the contrary, you've moved a great deal. You know so much more now,"Nacell declared. "Do you see the light straight ahead?" A rope of flame transformed the horizon.

"Is the water on fire?"

"On fire with energy, hope and joy," he smiled. "The color-scape ahead is comprised of salt lamps and salt candleholders."

Salt Secrets: Salt Tips for Life

Jasmine was not amused. "Lamps and candleholders do not float on water!"

"Yes, but these special lamps and candleholders are made of salt. Salt moves in water. Water conducts salt. And if you shine a flashlight on a salt crystal, you see the color the salt reflects," he said. Moreover, if you wish to view salt's true color, place the light behind the crystal." Nacell amplified his point by shining a light behind a salt lamp that was floating by.

"When light is reflected on an orange dress, the light you see appears as the color orange. But if you shine light behind the dress, the dress blocks the light.

"Salt transmits light. The atomic structure of salt allows light frequencies to move through it. Light is a source of life, and the sun is the major source of all natural light on the planet.

"Light brings heat and energy. Everyone has a relationship with light and is dependent on light. Without light, planet Earth would be a salty hunk of ice in no time at all. Yet, with all of your earthly

Salt Secrets: Salt Tips for Life

technologies and probing research, there is not a scientist on Earth who can explain exactly what light is." Nacell lowered his sunglasses for dramatic effect.

Jasmine was incredulous. "We can reach the moon, but scientists can't explain light?"

Nacell rolled up his proverbial sleeves, leaned forward and whispered: "No human has yet been able to see an electron. You can measure its presence, but even with an electron microscope, you cannot see an electron. Similarly, light is so small that no scientist has yet been able to see it. The truth of the color of light is not in your vocabulary," he declared.

"Most people do not realize that color is really a measure of the frequency of light – a reverberation or sympathetic vibration – and therefore the color you see depends on the frequency of that light.

"When the sound of music hits a certain frequency, we call it a note. By the same token, the name of a color is our best approximation for a frequency of light. But one doesn't say that a frequency is

Salt Secrets: Salt Tips for Life

breathtaking. Instead you exclaim: 'That color is breathtaking.' Some colors just sound right!" Nacell opined, waiting five seconds before he continued.

"When humans talk about emotions, they express them as colors. 'I'm in a blue mood.' 'I saw red.' 'He's green with envy.' Color affects your mood.

"Red is my favorite color," Jasmine announced.

"And that's why salt lamps and salt candleholders are energizing, yet calming. Indeed, many people are happiest when sleeping next to a lit salt lamp – whether the vibrant reddish orange hue of Himalayan or Polish salt lamps, the gentle blue of Persian salt lamps or earthier tones from South America.

"Orange relaxes the body. White has a detoxifying effect. Yellow activates the pancreas, liver and gall bladder. Pink stimulates emotions. Red activates the heart and helps blood circulation. Frequency hunger is akin to the nagging desire for a completely satisfying meal."

Salt Secrets: Salt Tips for Life

"I prefer to sleep in the dark," said Jasmine, "but yes, blue would be restful."

"Certain colors are calming, while others are stimulating," Nacell stated. "Humans are attracted to interesting forms of light – whether reflected, transmitted or projected. Colorful light affects their internal frequency in a positive way."

"Are you suggesting that human beings are built like radio waves?"

Nacell closed his eyes: "Yes, your internal frequency is also your internal light. Since light is a wave, your internal frequency can also be described as a wave. In fact, you're a virtual hotbed of frequencies. The gears of your brain are a frequency. Robin Williams, for example, has an especially high wit frequency brain; while many others I've met along the way haven't used their brain in years.

"Although time is a constant, some can complete more calculations per minute than others on a given topic. As you learn more about life, you think faster. Your pulse is a frequency: the number of times your heart

Salt Secrets: Salt Tips for Life

beats per minute. Blood pressure is based on the frequency of your heart beats.

"Human beings long for a connection to a higher frequency. They climb impossible mountains, parachute out of air planes and taking every possible risk to satisfy a need which often remains so elusive.

"Frequencies that move through salt crystals are filtered by the salt, resulting in purer colors – or a narrow range of frequencies. By isolating a certain frequency, salt lamps provide both an energetic and restful experience. You feel stimulated and yet in balance," he stressed.

"Crystals have been used to heal a variety of maladies for thousands of years. However, light that travels through a natural salt crystal – a mineral so essential for life – may be one of the most satisfying frequencies of all. Think of it as a 5-Star meal of light therapy for your body."

Jasmine was amazed. "In other words, salt lamps and salt candleholders make it easier to absorb light?"

Salt Secrets: Salt Tips for Life

"Precisely!" Nacell shimmered. "Just as the color of the salt lamp stimulates your eyes, it also stimulates a reaction from those hosts of frequencies within your body – bringing them into harmony. You might call it the perfect light salt diet!"

Salt Secrets: Salt Tips for Life

Exfoliate away your troubles! Combine one tablespoon of your best cognac with two tablespoons of organic olive oil, a quarter cup of artisan salt and five drops of essential lavender oil. Rub the solution all over your body. Rinse off with the purest mineral water you can find.

✭ Seven ✭

YOUR SALT BOAT

"**P**erfect harmony, like the perfect note, is impossible to sustain," he whispered. Once you experience internal balance, you want to feel it all of the time. And then, suddenly, you lose it.

"The body's awakening is akin to a lightning bolt. You might experience an epiphany that lasts for a split second. But if this is your initial glimpse of balance – if you're feeling a sublime stillness in your body for the first time – a second of perfection can be the event of a lifetime.

Draped across a wooden plank in the gently rocking boat, drinking in the sunlight, Jasmine found the cadence of Nacell's odd chatter strangely soothing.

"Just as the Primal Sea evaporated over time, your body could dry up for lack of harmony between the water and salt within you – that is, if you don't take care of your future in the present.

Salt Secrets: Salt Tips for Life

"So, for example, let's say that you decide to drink only one glass of water today – confident that you can drink three glasses tomorrow to bring yourself back to balance.

"By the second day, your body is convinced that you're in a drought. Even though you live in a modern society where you can easily obtain glass after glass of water, your body responds as if you're in desert-like conditions and starts conserving water.

"If you fail to hydrate on a continuous basis, your internal balance point will shift. Humans typically move further and further from their natural state of balance. Their bodies, lives and even their homes are facing a salt deficit."

"How can a home be in a salt deficit?"

Nacell grimaced. "The air within the average home is about five times more polluted than outdoor air, and Americans spend between sixty-five to ninety percent of their time indoors. Everyday activities like cleaning, cooking, heating, and cooling – and of course redecorating – release and spread indoor pollution.

Salt Secrets: Salt Tips for Life

"Home pollution includes bacteria, viruses, fungi, pollen, dust mites, animal dander and mold. These biological pollutants are often invisible, traveling through your home by air or via the surfaces you touch so many times a day." He feared that his remarks sounded like a college lecture. Yet, their hours together were fleeting, and there was so much vital information to impart."

"How do home pollutants end up in my body?" Jasmine asked.

"Either you inhale them directly or come in contact with polluted surfaces. They also settle on food and clothing. Subsequently, you touch your face or breathe them back into the air – resulting in allergic, infectious and even toxic reactions. The effects on your body are impossible to determine.

"Internally, your home craves balance and purity no less than you do. Instead, it's exposed to multiple toxins and myriads of chemical agents over lengthy periods. And that's where salt comes in. Natural salt home therapy can help provide a shield of protection for you and your beloved pet, Crystal."

Salt Secrets: Salt Tips for Life

Parodying a television newscaster, he went on: "Here's the great news! Salt crystals contain a unique mineral structure combining both sodium (positive) and chlorine (negative) ions. Negative ions help increase alertness and concentration. They also increase the lung's capacity to absorb oxygen while enhancing the respiratory tract's ability to deal with airborne particles. Negative ion emissions reduce a myriad of indoor air pollutants."

Pausing for effect, he went on: "Negative ions – or salt's negative side – alleviate common allergies and sinus conditions, depression caused by decreasing serotonin levels in the blood stream, sleep disorders, migraine headaches, flu susceptibility and bronchial problems, including asthma. They remove toxic substances from the home by reducing biological contaminants, including pollen germs, bacteria, mold, mildew, dust mites and animal dander. They can also help remove odor and smoke, enhance your immune system, increase alertness and concentration, and reduce hormonal imbalances."

Nacell was out of breath. Jasmine was intrigued, but concerned. As a home-based entrepreneur, the specter of all of this dirt inside her condo was more than she could bear. "It sounds awful. What can I possibly do about it?"

"Turn on a salt lamp. It's better to light a single salt lamp than curse the dirt!" Nacell chuckled.

"Use a salt lamp to fight indoor pollution?" Jasmine pursued her lips. Wouldn't the lamp be just another dust collector?"

"Yes, that's precisely the beauty of natural salt crystal lamps and natural salt crystal candleholders," Nacell reverberated. "Imbued with negative ions, they act as natural air purifiers or natural ionizers by removing toxic particles from the air.

"Negative ions contain an extra electron – also called a static charge – that is just waiting to jump ship. The negative ion's extra electron can only escape if it locates and attaches itself to a positive or neutral particle floating in the air.

"The newly created clump is heavier and therefore tends to drift to the ground – splat, right on the floor! You can then vacuum or mop up the toxic or dusty clump," Nacell explained. "I suggest that you use a

Salt Secrets: Salt Tips for Life

mop, because as we all know, nature abhors a vacuum. When you turn on a salt lamp, extra electrons are generated, which then dance on the surface of the lamp waiting for particles to come by. Heat generated by the light bulb – or by a candle placed inside a salt candleholder – warms the air.

"Hot air rises. As the artificially generated salt ions rise with the hot air, they increase air circulation, remove dust and reduce humidity in the air."

"In other words, negative ions have positive benefits!" Jasmine smiled at her play on words. "What about regular candles? Do they clean the air as well?"

"Paraffin candles are made from a petroleum by-product that releases soot," he replied. Mentally counting the number of wax candles in her living room, Jasmine was pensive.

"Salt helps restore energy and balance in your home in numerous ways," Nacell added. "Feng Shui experts, for example, sprinkle salt around the perimeter of the room to erase negative energy and to create a positive perimeter of wealth. I met

Salt Secrets: Salt Tips for Life

a famous princess thousand of years ago who cleaned every corner of her castle with salt."

Jasmine couldn't envision her cluttered apartment as a castle.

"You readily accepted that you're in a wooden boat," Nacell diverted to another stream of thought. "But on closer examination, you will see that the boat is made of salt."

She jolted upright. How could her boat possibly be made of salt?

"This boat is an outcropping of salt from ancient waters that receded over the ages," he said, but immediately changed the subject.

Salt Secrets: Salt Tips for Life

Salt is contrary. It comes from water, but makes you thirsty. It corrodes metal, but preserves your food. Salt is hard, yet softens your food.

✷ Eight ✷

YOUR SALT CAVE

"Do you know what salt smells like?" Nacell inquired. "The lack of anything has a crisp smell of its own. Have you ever actually smelled salt?"

Jasmine was offended. "How can nothing have a smell? And yes, I can easily smell salt at the sea shore."

Nacell offered a wry smile. "If you ask people what they like most about the sea shore, the majority will insist that they love the smell of salt. Yet, what they smell is actually a combination of moss, mold, kelp, silicon and dead fish, combined with the cleansing characteristics of salt in the air. In other words, they smell the many inclusions in the sea shore environment, but not the salt."

Nacell attempted to sniff the air. "Here's a glass of water with a teaspoon of table salt and another

Salt Secrets: Salt Tips for Life

glass with only water. Can you smell the difference?" He handed Jasmine two glasses of water.

Jasmine frowned. "There's no difference."

"But surely you can see a difference between the water in the two glasses?" he persisted.

"Yes, the water in the second glass is cloudy."

Nacell appeared to be juggling two bright red tomatoes. "If I hand you a tomato with salt on it and a tomato without salt, you will have difficulty perceiving a difference."

He was building up to a peak moment. "Look around. What do you smell?" Nacell flashed a light on the walls of what seemed to be a cave.

Jasmine was horrified. "When did we enter a cave?"

Nacell quickly pulled out a small capsule of smelling salts and floated it under her nose. "This is my cousin, smelling salts. Though he smells like

Salt Secrets: Salt Tips for Life

ammonia, he's really a salt. A colorless-to-white crystalline solid salt called Aromatic Spirits of Ammonia or Ammonium Carbonate, to be precise. He'll awaken your senses."

"I do not want salt that smells like ammonia, my senses are just fine, and I demand that you explain why you took me to a cave." She brushed the smelling salts to the ground.

Elated by her anger, Nacell replied: "Now, in a perfectly dry salt cave that hasn't been disturbed in years, you cannot smell much. You might smell other elements found in the cave, but not the salt. That's because salt in a solid form does not transmit much of a scent.

"When water and salt molecules collide in the ocean, numerous salt particles are also tossed up into the air. The only time you detect molecular salt in the air is when these tiny salt particles enter your nose.

"It's often said that ninety percent of taste is in the nose. While your nose sensors detect the physical presence of salt, the salt particles are so small that

Salt Secrets: Salt Tips for Life

you rarely smell salt on its own, that is, without inclusions. Pure salts are non-volatile and odorless, while salt inclusions have an aroma when activated or released. Smelling salts, for example, smell like ammonia."

"Would you like something to eat?" Nacell pointed to a table overflowing with Jasmine's favorite foods. Each was adorned by a tiny flag listing the salt content. How could a piece of cake include so much salt, she wondered? The doughnut was off the salt charts. Her favorite coffee, Happy Meal and to-die-for pastrami sandwich all had huge amounts of salt.

"How can sweet or spicy food possibly contain so much salt?"

"Oh, but I am sweet," Nacell insisted, "Just as food can be sweet and sour, it can also be salty and sweet. Hidden salt makes food tasty and can even be addictive. One donut isn't harmful, though a half might be better. It's all about moderation. The dinner bell rings not for salt, but for salt solutions."

Salt Secrets: Salt Tips for Life

Nacell recalled that diamonds are a girl's best friend. Hoping to change the tempo, he said, "Salt crystals were called the King's Diamond in ancient times.

"Alexander the Great discovered the healing powers of salt caves during his battles in India. Fighting on scorching plains by day, his troops sought shelter in ancient Himalayan salt caves by night. The wounds suffered by both men and horses sheltered in the caves healed rapidly and beyond expectation. His troops also demonstrated stronger endurance during battle. Alexander concluded that the pure salt found there had curative powers.

"He ordered his men to begin mining the salt crystals, and salt soon became a prized currency. Indeed, the word 'salary' derives from salt, while salarium argentum means 'salt money' in Latin. Men who worked in salt mines were frequently paid in salt. To this day, hard work is equated with working in a salt mine."

Jasmine felt increasingly tranquil inside the cave. In spite of her trepidation, she was also growing

Salt Secrets: Salt Tips for Life

fond of Nacell and his peculiar tales. Glancing about, she saw no way in or out. Oddly, the lack of an apparent exit didn't worry her. Taking an especially deep breath, she decided to simply enjoy the present.

Nacell elaborated: "Salt cave therapy, also known as Speleotherapy, is available in many countries, including Austria, Rumania, Poland, Azerbaijan and the Ukraine. Halite dust (natural dry sodium chloride suspended in air), which charges the air and changes its texture, is the primary healing factor.

"The comfortable cave climate – free of humidity and allergens – reinforces the healing process, while the concentration of carbon dioxide induces deeper and more intensive breathing. You can also enjoy salt cave therapy without leaving the country. Halotherapy simulates the natural microclimate of a salt cave. It is performed in a special room with salt-coated walls and floors. Dry halite is released into the room."

Nacell held a smoking pipe in his hand. Jasmine fretted that he would ruin her glorious salt cave

Salt Secrets: Salt Tips for Life

experience by lighting up tobacco. "Salt pipes and saline devices are also therapeutic for respiratory problems," Nacell explained, pouring salt into the pipe. For the first time during her journey, Jasmine was able to laugh at her qualms.

He noted her turning point. "Though you may not smell cave salt, it nevertheless envelopes you in a sense of serenity once attainable only by the wealthy. There are numerous forms of wealth, including the money-wealth you've been chasing, health-wealth which you lack and the fleeting wealth of internal balance.

"The path to health is a life choice. Those who seek out salt therapies, like so many other forms of therapy, are acknowledging that their lives could be better. The best way to determine if a particular type of salt can energize or rebalance your life is to include it in your daily regimen and see if you notice any changes."

Nacell drew himself up to his full height, adopted his best Brad Pitt demeanor and looked penetratingly into Jasmine's eyes. "Jasmine, can you hear the sound of salt?"

Salt Secrets: Salt Tips for Life

She was startled by the question.

"The sound of salt depends on whether salt is putting out a wave. If you pour a teaspoon of natural salt into a glass jar, you might hear a whooshing sound – and if you listen closely, you can even hear salt hit the side of the glass.

"Salt rarely makes a noise by itself; instead, it reacts with its environment. The real secret is whether you hear the sound of salt resonating within your own body."

✶ Nine ✶

YOUR SALT SPA

"Do you know how much salt there is in seawater?"

"I haven't the foggiest idea," Jasmine responded.

"It's a question few think about and yet almost seventy-five percent of the world lives by the sea or within the ocean's ecosystem. If you were to fill a quart container with seawater, it would weigh about 1,000 grams. Remove just the water from the container and what's left behind will weigh roughly 35 grams — 85.6 percent of which is salt — or a total of about 30 grams of sodium chloride or table salt. The sodium and chlorine atoms composing the 30 grams of salt are not present in equal amounts.

"Chlorine, which is heavier, represents about 60 percent of the 30 grams. These 30 grams of salt contain almost 18 grams of chlorine and 12 grams of sodium, plus tiny amounts of other materials.

Salt Secrets: Salt Tips for Life

Of course your result may vary depending on the time of day, depth of water or who just swam by."

Nacell gave a salty laugh. "The ocean is your body's mirror, and your body is actually a living seawater bath. Take 100 gallons of seawater; mix in a few other vital minerals found in the ocean, add heat, light and a pinch of just about anything else and voila! You have the initial ingredients to create a person, though it will take a few million years. And speaking of salt baths, would you like to visit our Primal Sea Salt Spa?"

"A spa in the middle of the Primal Sea?" Jasmine's heart skipped a beat.

"Yes, we have a lovely salt spa. Unfortunately, it's a long walk. If you're not up to it... "

Jasmine bolted forward. "Just point the way sir gallant salt!" Before she knew it, they were standing under an immense waterfall – though not a drop touched her. A colorful sign read: "Welcome to the Primal Sea Salt Spa.'

Salt Secrets: Salt Tips for Life

"Cleopatra would be envious," Nacell remarked, admiring Jasmine's attire. Looking at her reflection in the water, Jasmine was shocked to discover that she was cloaked in a huge white terry cloth robe. A gleaming white tub stood directly in her path.

Nacell bowed. "I'll be waiting in the lobby, my lady." And then he vanished.

An emerald tray with a small flowering Jasmine plant levitated next to the tub. A tantalizing assortment of natural salt skin care items surrounded the plant, including salt cleansing bars, salt facial and body scrubs, salt mud masks and salt lotions. Luxuriating in the salty bath water, Jasmine was ecstatic. It felt like paradise on earth.

The salt cleansing bar slipped out of her hand and skipped along the top of the water. Jasmine giggled, splashed about and felt better than she had in years. Holding the salt bar, she gently moved it down her arms. She loved the tingling sensation, so silky to the touch. Next she tried the facial scrub and then applied a thick salt clay mask.

Salt Secrets: Salt Tips for Life

Tension evaporated from every muscle in her body. Jasmine had a sudden flashback to the first time her dad took her to an amusement park, showering her with attention, roller coaster rides and cotton candy. It was their magical day together. And this was her magical day – a roller coaster ride, to be sure, but full of sweet surprises.

Clashing cymbals ruined her reverie. "Your coach has arrived!" Nacell trumpeted in a deep voice. "Please watch your step."

A mirror-paneled coach stood before her. Jasmine's favorite old faded robe hung from the door facing her. But there were no horses in sight, and her glorious salt spa had vanished. She was terribly upset. "Must we leave now?"

"The drape will be opening soon," Nacell declared, making little sense. "You must get your beauty sleep."

"But I'm not tired. I feel so invigorated."

"All things in balance," said Nacell. "It's best to start early if you don't want to be late." Jasmine

Salt Secrets: Salt Tips for Life

entered the coach with a heavy heart. A small ruby-colored pouch was on the opposite seat.

"It's a gift," said Nacell, turning away shyly.

Opening the pouch slowly to savor the surprise, Jasmine discovered a reddish orange salt crystal pendant. The salt crystal was artisan wrapped in delicate gold wire and suspended from a thin golden thread.

"I hope you will...that you might...think of me when you wear it," Nacelle spoke gently. For the first time since they met, he stumbled over his words.

"It is absolutely precious," said Jasmine, touched by Nacell's kindness and by his sudden bashfulness. She slipped the salt pendant over her head, fascinated by the myriad points of reflected light.

Nacell felt his throat tighten: "Jasmine, I hope this pendant reminds you of the special salt journey that we shared. I will be listening for your salt vibration until the end of time." He stared off into the distance to regain his composure. The coach came to a sudden stop.

"But now the hour has arrived for your salt boudoir," he said, pointing to a regal salt chamber just ahead. The floor and walls were tiled with mesmerizing salt tablets. "You can't imagine how soothing a natural salt night can be. Would you like a salt blanket and a salt pillow?"

Jasmine wasn't ready to retire or to take leave of Nacell. He had struck a deep emotional chord, and she was only beginning to understand him. A salty tear rushed down her cheek.

"Just a short nap," she reluctantly agreed. Pulling the salt blanket over her shoulder, Jasmine turned on her side to nestle into the luxurious salt pillow.

At that very moment, Crystal leapt onto the bed, mewing urgently into Jasmine's ear. Jasmine was ecstatic. "Nacell promised that you were waiting for me!"

But where was her salt boudoir? As the room came into focus, Jasmine found herself staring at

Salt Secrets: Salt Tips for Life

framed photographs of her mom and dad, prized knickknacks and a pile of long-delayed paperwork.

How did she end up back in her own bedroom? It was only a dream after all. Nacell didn't exist. What a fool she was to believe for even a second that he was real.

Slowly swinging her legs over the side of the bed, Jasmine walked dejectedly to the window, pulling the drape on a new day. Several seconds rushed by before she noticed the reddish orange frequency reflected in the glass. A beautiful salt crystal pendant artistically wrapped in a delicate gold wire adorned her neck.

Salt Secrets: Salt Tips for Life

Afterword

Jasmine moved to an apartment by the seashore, where she listens for Nacell's vibration above the waves. Actively pursuing salt health and salt beauty regimes, she watches her salt intake and only eats the type of salt that her body really needs. She also keeps salt lamps and salt candleholders in every room. Friends comment that her skin is aglow and that her home is so restful.

Jasmine's life is finally in balance. Feeling healthier and more energized, her creativity has soared, and she's virtually flooded with fascinating graphic art assignments. She's also begun carving an artistic niche in the medium of salt.

Nacell finds himself yearning for Jasmine's human vibration. He tries to overcome this unfamiliar pain by steeping himself in plans to receive the next salt seeker at the Natural Salt Oasis. Are you ready to take the journey?

SECTION II

SALT WEALTH TIPS FOR BODY, SPIRIT AND HOME

Salt Secrets: Salt Tips for Life

✳ Ten ✳

SALT TIPS FOR LIFE

Natural mineral edible salts tend to have a distinctive taste and can greatly enhance your meal. They also include a variety of minerals that help the body remain in balance. However, adding naturally occurring salt to a daily regime of excess salt could destabilize your health. Choose the source of your healing salt wisely and for the purpose at hand.

The vast majority of men and women ingest more salt than they need. According to the National Academy of Sciences (NAS), the average adult requires 2300 milligrams grams of salt daily or approximately one teaspoon of salt. Indeed, the USDA recommends that certain groups, including Blacks and the elderly, consume no more 1500 milligrams of salt each day.

Hidden Salt: Salt is a combination of two natural elements: sodium and chlorine. Food labels

Salt Secrets: Salt Tips for Life

typically list sodium rather than salt content. A food item is low in salt if it has less than less than 140 mg or five percent of the Daily Value [DV] in sodium. Sodium content can also vary by several hundreds of milligrams in similar foods. Sodium used by manufacturers to preserve food items accounts for almost 80 percent of the salt intake for most people – while natural occurring salt accounts for only 10 percent and edible salt for another five to 10 percent of their total intake.

Salt You Need: To ensure that the salt you ingest is the salt you need: 1) Consult with your doctor before ingesting high quantities of any salt product; 2) Read the label to determine which minerals and elements are included; 3) Experiment with different types of salt until you find the salt that your body needs.

Salt Vitamin Drink: The salt vitamin drink – Salt Solution – has been popular in Europe for decades. There is some confusion between the original name of this drink – often referred to as Sol or Sole´ (soleil is the French sun) – and companies that later branded these terms with their business name. A rock crystal by any other

Salt Secrets: Salt Tips for Life

name is still a rock. The challenge is to find a reputable supplier of the highest grade edible Himalayan salt and <u>edible Himalayan salt chunks</u>.

<u>Please be on notice</u>: A foreign facility that exports edible salt – or any other edible product – to the United States must register with the FDA, whereas a foreign facility that exports salt chunks for bathing is not required to register with the FDA. Be certain that you purchase high-grade edible salt chunks for the salt vitamin drink.

"High-grade Himalayan salt is harvested from salt veins in the mountain," explained Naomi Novotny, vice president of SaltWorks, Inc. (www.saltworks.com).

"However, some companies collect and sell debris that is leftover from main salt mining expeditions. Others mine low-grade deposits from other parts of the Mountain, but claim the salt is edible. A foreign supplier that exports bath salts, versus edible salts, does not require FDA clearance. The distributor should also provide assurances that the salt has been carefully screened for unwanted inclusions (like dirt and other foreign particles)."

Salt Secrets: Salt Tips for Life

Although salt is a natural antibiotic, you can't be certain how many hands have touched the chunks along the supply route. Gently wash your salt chunks with purified or distilled water before using them in a salt vitamin drink.

Here are the steps for preparing your Salt Solution: Select a <u>few</u> (two or three) rock crystal salt chunks and place them in a tightly capped, medium sized glass jar. Pour high quality mineral water (approximately 4-5 ounces) into the jar. A small instant coffee glass jar works perfectly. Let the salt brine solution stand overnight. The water is salt saturated when the crystals stop dissolving and only a few small crystals remain at the bottom of the jar. Mix one <u>teaspoon</u> of the solution in an eight-ounce glass of pure mineral water and drink before breakfast.

Salt Solution 'devotees' often report that their energy levels have soared – yet their daily vitamin intake has decreased. One devotee wrote: "My body feels so balanced. I was taking supplements with high trace mineral content for energy that cost me about $30 to $40 dollars a month. Now, I

Salt Secrets: Salt Tips for Life

only take a teaspoon each morning, and I am ready to go!"

Again, please do not use MORE of this brine solution than your body requires. New users have been known to mix several tablespoons of brine solution into a glass of water, rather than a single teaspoon! This could result in a greater salt intake than your body can readily absorb! Moderation is essential. Further, as Nacell points out, those who suffer from inner ear problems should carefully moderate the amount of salt they absorb for any purpose – including salt baths! Women who are pregnant or nursing should be extremely careful of inclusions in any salt they ingest.

Artisan Salt: Discover the exotic power of edible artisan salts. Season your culinary canvas with salts from around the world, including: Alaea Hawaiin Sea Salt, Bolivian Rose, Cyprus Black Lava (salt combined with charcoal), Flor de Sal from Portugal, Flower of Bali, Himalayan Pink Salt, India Black Salt, Sel de Mer from the Mediterranean, Pure Ocean Atlantic Sea Salt from Brazil and Sel Gris (harvested through Celtic methods). Food will never taste quite the same.

Salt Secrets: Salt Tips for Life

Salt was used long before people started writing things down. Even so, salt is mentioned in the Chinese publication Peng-Tzao-Kan-Mu, written about 2700 BC. This work contains the earliest known treatise on pharmacology, [including] the details on more than forty kinds of salt.

"In West Africa on the southern edge of the Sahara desert, empires were built on the salt trade. In some trading cities in this region (like the famous Timbuktu) salt could be traded ounce-for-ounce for gold.

– www.ChemHeritage.org

✫ Eleven ✫

SALT TIPS TO REDUCE MUSCLE TENSION AND STRESS

Dead Sea salt, Epsom salts and Himalayan salt crystals are among the most effective for reducing muscle tension and daily stress. Experts recommend that your salt bath water be lukewarm and that you remain for at least twenty minutes.

Salt Healing for Soft Tissue Injuries: I was in an elevator accident in the late 1990s. Spending untold sums on a variety of therapeutic treatments, the pain always returned. However, once I began to bathe daily in Himalayan salt, to wrap my neck in a towel soaked in Himalayan salt crystals and to drink the salt solution daily, the pain slowly evaporated. Himalayan salt seemed to help my body heal itself.

A colleague also told me the following story: His eight-year-old son took a fall that left him hopping on one foot. The pain in the boy's right foot was excruciating. The parents tried numerous remedies over several days, but nothing seemed to help. The father then recalled what I told him about my own salt experiments. He wrapped his son's foot in a towel soaked with Himalayan salt water. His son was back on both feet in a matter of hours and suffered no further pain.

Another word of caution: If the pain in your neck or back subsides, don't take unnecessary risks and injure yourself once again. The injured area remains vulnerable.

Salt Healing for Heal Spurs: Heel spur calcifications form as a result of damage to the plantar fascia. Magnesium transports calcium out of your body. Frequent bathing in natural mineral Epsom Salt helps breaks down heal spur calcifications and remove them from the body.

Salt Breathing: 'Speleo' is Greek for cave. Caves were viewed as healing environments even in ancient times. Animals also retreat to caves to heal wounds or stings. In 1843, Polish physician F. Bochkowsky postulated that air saturated with

Salt Secrets: Salt Tips for Life

saline dust is the primary curative effect in the speleotherapy of patients with respiratory diseases. During the Second World War, villagers across Eastern Europe often hid in salt caves or salt mines for long periods. According to numerous reports, coughs, colds and other maladies were soon alleviated or disappeared completely.

Substantial scientific research has not been undertaken. However, on one of the first systematic studies undertaken on asthma, daily four-hour treatments for a period of six to eight weeks reportedly resulted in improvements lasting six months to seven years (Skulimowski, 1965).

Halotherapy: You can also simulate the natural salt cave microclimate in your own home through halo healing chambers. Halotherapy involves dry salt aerosol inhalation. HT is performed in a special room with salt-coated walls and floor - the Halochamber. Dry sodium chloride aerosol containing particles 1-5um in size is produced by a special nebulizer and released into the Halochamber, (www.HaloTherapy.com).

Salt Secrets: Salt Tips for Life

From magnesium chloride, the Dead Sea Works also produces magnesium, a metal that is seven times stronger than steel and lighter than aluminum.

– Mark Kulansky, *SALT*

☆ Twelve ☆

SALT TIPS FOR UPLIFTING YOUR SPIRITS WITH VIVID DECOR

Salt lamps, salt candleholders and salt tiles provide vivid color therapy for home and spirit. Featuring orange, white, yellow, pink and reddish hues, these earth-given products foster a restful, yet energizing environment. Orange soothes the nervous system. White has a detoxifying effect. Yellow activates the pancreas, liver and gall bladder. Pink stimulates emotions. Red activates the heart and blood circulation.

Salt candleholders are comparative in price to the most popular decor candles – but with many additional benefits. The deep inner recess for a small tealight candle reduces the dangers of flying sparks. The tealight flame burns well below the top of the candleholder. Use a scented tealight for salt crystal aroma therapy!

Salt Secrets: Salt Tips for Life

You can also place a few drops of essential oil directly on the lamp. If the scent is too powerful, wipe the area with a slightly damp cloth until the aroma is just right. Why purchase costly aroma therapy dispensers when your lamp can do the job for free?

Keep your salt lamps lit at all times for the continuous color therapy and air purification results. The bulb amplifies air ionization, purification and detoxification by stimulating the production of healthy "negative" salt ions. Each lamp requires only four watts of electricity (the standard night bulb), although some users prefer 15 watt bulbs for maximum benefit.

The bulb is easily replaced and can be purchased from any pharmacy or grocery store. Salt lamps that remain lit can also help decrease electricity costs, since you are less likely to flip the switch for overhead lights every time you enter the room. Pack a small lamp – or several candleholders – for hotel stays. Purify that musty hotel air.

Heat from tealight candle also stimulates the release of negative ions. The candleholder purifies

Salt Secrets: Salt Tips for Life

the air without a candle - just more slowly. By contrast, electric candles deplete negative ions, while battery operated candles produce environmental contamination when you dispose of the batteries. Wax candles do not generate negative ions and therefore cannot purify the air.

Salt Decor

Salt lamps and salt candleholders vary in size and quality. Be certain that the seller or the seller's distributor has <u>tested the product</u>. "We put our products through a rigorous six-step quality assurance test," said Gerald Katen, managing director of the Black Tai Salt Company (www.BlackTaiSaltCo.com), a leading global distributor of salt lamps, salt candleholders and exotic bath salts.

"The testing process covers height, thickness, appearance, moisture content and possible cracks. We also test each lamp to ensure a solid wooden base," Katen explained.

Salt Secrets: Salt Tips for Life

Salt lamps and candleholders can be deployed throughout your home:

Entry Foyer: Greet guests with healing art.
Living Room: Feature next to your couch.
Dining Room: Dine by the light of the sea.
Den: Counter harmful television rays.
Bedrooms: Use as bedside lamps.
Kitchen: Diffuse microwave rays and odors.
Home Office: Counter electro-smog.

Salt tiled walls and floors are increasingly popular in spas and restaurants around the world. Enhance a wall or floor of your home with stunning and restful salt tiles.

While the lamps and candleholders will not lose their shape, the vivid colors might fade if left in intense sunlight over a prolonged period. Use a red or orange light bulb to help restore the luster.

If you drop or break your lamp or candleholder, simply hammer it into pieces and use the salt chips for cleaning purposes, as a small hand soap or as Feng Shui space clearing crystals. (Do not use

Salt Secrets: Salt Tips for Life

broken lamp or candleholder chips to prepare your Salt Solution vitamin drink!)

<u>If your home is highly humid:</u> If your home is humid and the lamps remain off for lengthy periods, moisture will likely form on the exterior. In such cases, it's best not to place a lamp close to your computer or other electrical appliance.

Saltwater intrusion will harm your computer. Keep the lamp at least a foot away. Candleholders can also be placed in a shallow bowl or dish, rather than directly on a glass or wood surface. If salty water forms, use the residue as a cleaning solution. It's an excellent way to recycle.

All lamps and candleholders should be wiped at least monthly with a dry cloth to remove dust or other particles.

Salt Secrets: Salt Tips for Life

Salt has fascinated man for thousands of years as a generator of poetic and of mythic meaning. The contradictions it embodies only intensify its power and its links with experience of the sacred.

– Margaret Visser, Author

☆ Thirteen ☆

SALT TIPS FOR FACE & BODY

Natural artisan salt is used in a wide array of revitalizing beauty products, including facial cleansers and tightening masks; face creams, body creams, hand creams, and natural soaps, as well as salt therapy eye masks and pillows that can be stored in the freezer or heated in the oven.

But why spend money on pricey salt therapy products when you can create your own solutions for a fraction of the price? For best results, use finely granulated Himalayan salt crystals, Dead Sea salt, Epsom salts, Celtic salt or other premier artisan salts.

Salt Facial Scrubs: Create a healthy glow with a homemade salt facial scrub. Combine one tablespoon of healthy salt with one tablespoon of olive oil and/or with a tablespoon of honey. Gently massage over your skin in a circular motion. Avoid the delicate under-eye area. Leave the 'olive oil honey salt mask' on your face for at least 20 minutes. Olive oil and honey soften skin, while salt absorbs the excess oil. Salt also polishes away dead skin cells, leaving a radiant complexion and wonderful skin tone.

Salt Lemon Lavender Bath Scrub: Place three or four teaspoons of healing salt in a small cosmetic jar. Add enough lemon juice to cover the salt. Add three or four drops of essential Lavender oil. Mix well. Gently scrub the solution over your entire body. Don't forget your feet! Lemon is a light acid and therefore a great exfoliating agent. Lemon juice is also a powerful detoxifying agent that can draw the toxins out of your body through your skin and feet. Keep your feet raised for about 10 minutes if possible. Shower or bathe off the residue. Go to sleep immediately following this blissful Lemon Lavender Salt Scrub experience. You will be so refreshed when you awaken that you will feel as if you just took a spa vacation.

Caution: Consult with your doctor prior to taking an Epsom salt bath if you have high blood pressure, heart problems, or if you are diabetic.

Salt Secrets: Salt Tips for Life

Salt Rubdown: While still in the tub, or just before stepping out of the tub – while your skin is still damp – massage yourself with a handful of natural mineral salt.

Salt Skin Purifier: Salt cleansing bars are wonderful detoxifying alternatives to processed soap containing aluminium salt, alcohol or perfume. Salt bars do not leave a soapy (mildew generating) residue, nor do they stain clothing. Use the salt bar to wash your face, body and hands and to stimulate your scalp. Take care that the bar is completely smooth with no rough surfaces. Possible "inclusions" might scratch your skin. If the salt bar is not completely smooth, use a wash cloth instead. Wet the bar and use the salty residue on the cloth.

Salt Skin Softener: Dissolve one cup of your favorite healing salt in a tub and soak as usual. Your entire body will feel noticeably softer. Add a few drops of pure essential oil and/or herbal tea bags for an especially soothing treatment.

Salt Secrets: Salt Tips for Life

Salt for Dandruff, Blisters and Stings

Salt Away Dandruff: Your skin contains a variety of oils. Dandruff appears when skin is sloughed or scratched for any reason. When it comes from the top of your head, it's called dandruff. The abrasiveness of Himalayan salt helps remove both dander and dandruff. Shake a bit of finely granulated Himalayan salt onto your dry scalp and massage it into your hair before you shampoo.

Salt for Blisters & Poison Ivy: Mix one teaspoon of salt in one cup of water. Soak a cotton pad in the salt water and apply to the affected area. The antiseptic properties of salt help reduce inflammation. Poison Ivy itching can also be reduced by soaking the affected area in hot salty water.

Salt for Stings: Salt reduces pain and swelling. For relief of mosquito and chigger bites, soak the area in salt water, then apply a coating of Crisco or vegetable oil.

Salt Deodorizers

Deodorizer: Salt cleansing bars leave an invisible layer of protection that helps prevent the formation of odor-causing bacteria. Wet the stone and glide it slowly over your underarm area. However, as noted above, if there are jagged edges that can scratch your skin, slide a washcloth across the bar instead. Avoid direct contact.

Garlic: Remove garlic smells from your hands by rubbing your fingers with salt.

Hand-Soap: Salt bars created from a variety of pure edible food products or carved directly from their natural surroundings combat bacteria without side-affects. And don't throw away those extra chips. I wash my hands daily with chunks from a broken salt candleholder. Keep extra salt pieces in a dish for a quick hand-wash or to purify your kitchen and bathroom air! If you break a salt lamp or salt candleholder, recycle!

Salt Secrets: Salt Tips for Life

Salt Oral Care

Salt Oral Care: Use natural edible salt as a substitute for costly toothpastes. Your teeth will gleam, and your gums will appreciate the gentle but effective treatment. Place finely-ground natural salt on your toothbrush or use some of your Salt Solution. For a quick breath freshener, mix one teaspoon edible salt and one teaspoon baking soda into a half cup of water. Rinse and gargle. Add a few drops of essential peppermint oil for flavor.

Salt Energy Gemstones

Crystals have been used in healing for thousands of years. Himalayan salt crystals can be worn as healing gemstones. They have the same structure as diamonds – octahedrons or eight-sided figures – while the beautiful colors are based on reflected and refracted light.

Salt Secrets: Salt Tips for Life

The Himalayan Primal Sea Salt Crystal Energy Pendant ™ – designed and created by this author in 2006 – is an artisan-crafted remnant of the earth's original Primal Sea. Energizing salt pendants are artistically wrapped in polished silver or gold wire to protect the delicate salt crystal. Each is hand-crafted according to the unique shape of the crystal.

With stunning angled shapes and hues, the Himalayan Primal Sea Crystal Energy Pendant™ is a true healing original.

Energy Pendants are offered exclusively on www.Dr.JoyceStarr.com and on websites owned by Dr. Starr. They can also be ordered by phone at: 1-786-693-4223.

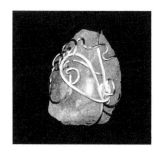

Salt Secrets: Salt Tips for Life

There is sufficient salt in the seas of our planet to wrap the world in a 147-foot layer of salt.

⋆ Fourteen ⋆

SALT TIPS FOR YOUR KITCHEN

You can use many types of salt for both food preparation and kitchen cleansing, including Celtic Salt, Himalayan Salt, Kosher Salt, Mediterranean Salt and Morton's Salt. Choose the salt that best fits your purpose and budget.

The word salt connotes 'neutral.' Salt is neither an acid nor a base, so it will not strip or harm most surfaces.

Salt is also physically gritty. When moved across a surface, it destabilizes the bond with grime. Twenty-two thousand substances qualify as home grime.

Salt is a chemical-free cleansing agent. Use it for floor tiles, kitchen counters and bathroom sinks to fight bacteria and add sparkle to your home.

Salt Secrets: Salt Tips for Life

Salt Tips for Food Preparation

You can use artisan salt or ordinary table salt for all of the tips below.

Cheese: Wrap cheese in a cloth napkin soaked in salt water to prevent molding.

Coffee: Add a touch of salt to the brew to sweeten your coffee.

Cooking: Add a pinch or two of salt to boiling water to reduce cooking time. Salt helps water boil at a higher temperature.

Crispy Salad: Add a touch of salt to your salad immediately after preparation. It should remain crisp for several hours.

Dough: Wiping up dough with water and sponge just makes it worse! Sprinkle the area with salt and rub with a barely damp cloth. This will help avoid a sticky mess.

Salt Secrets: Salt Tips for Life

Fruit: Soak apples and pears in lightly salted water to prevent browning. Smoothen the skin of older fruit by soaking the fruit in lightly salted water.

Milk: Add a pinch of salt to a gallon of milk to keep it fresher and longer.

Pecans: Soak pecans in salt water for several hours before shelling. The pecan meat will separate easily from the shells.

Sugaring, Crazing and Cracking: Add a pinch of salt to cake icing to prevent crystallization.

Vegetables: Mix a tablespoon of salt in a quart of filtered water. Rinse your vegetables several times with the solution.

Whipping Cream: Add a pinch of salt to whipping cream to beat faster and higher.

Salt Secrets: Salt Tips for Life

Salt Tips for Eggs

Fresh Eggs: Add two teaspoons of salt to one cup of water. Gently place eggs in the cup. Fresh eggs will sink, while older eggs will float.

Peeling Hard-Boiled Eggs: Add a teaspoon of salt to the pot before boiling. The eggs will be easier to shell.

Poached Eggs: Sprinkle a half teaspoon of salt into the water before cooking to even the edges of poached eggs.

Whipped Eggs: Add a pinch of salt to the egg mixture. It will beat more easily.

Salt Tips for Cooking Ware & Glasses

Bacon Grease: Add a few dashes of salt to the pan before frying foods that can splatter.

Baked-On Food: Stop scrubbing baked-on food from plates or casseroles. Sprinkle a bit of salt on

Salt Secrets: Salt Tips for Life

the dish, dampen with water and let it set for a couple of hours. Food will wash away easily.

Burned Milk: Burned milk is almost impossible to remove, but salt makes it easier. Wet the burned pan and sprinkle it with salt. Wait about 10 minutes and then scrub the pan. Salt absorbs the bad odor as well.

Cast Iron: Sprinkle salt in a greasy cast-iron pan before you wash it. Many old-timers scrub the pan with salt before adding water. Salt absorbs most of the grease. Wipe the pan and then wash as usual.

Enamel Pans: Enamel pans often cook stains right into the surface. Rather than scrubbing to no avail, just soak overnight in a solution of water and a half cup of salt. Boil your enamel pan in the salty water the following day. Stains should rinse off easily.

Discolored glasses: You don't have to buy expensive dishwasher aids to remove spots from your glasses. Just mix a handful of salt in a quart of vinegar and soak the glasses overnight. Stains should wipe off easily in the morning.

Salt Secrets: Salt Tips for Life

Lipstick Marks on Glasses: Before washing your glassware, rub the edges with salt to erase lipstick stains.

Oven and Stove-top Spills: If food bubbles over in your oven, immediately sprinkle salt on the spill while it is still liquid. When the oven cools, wipe up the spill with a cloth. You can also clean stove-top spills with salt.

Refrigerator: Use one-quarter cup salt in a two-liter bottle of warm water to wash all inner and outer surfaces of your fridge. This is effective, quick, nontoxic and gives the fridge a clean crisp smell.

Spilt Eggs: Cover the spill with salt. It will draw the egg together and you can easily wipe them up with a sponge or paper towel.

Tea and Coffee Stains on Cups: Scrub stains away with salt of almost any variety. Just sprinkle salt on a sponge and rub in little circles across the ring. If the stain doesn't go disappear, mix white vinegar and salt in equal proportions and rub with the sponge.

Salt Secrets: Salt Tips for Life

Teapots: Fill the teapot with salty water until the water rises to the spout. Let it sit overnight. Then run boiling water through the pot, washing away the salt. If the stain persists, rub the rim with a cotton swab dipped in salt.

Wood Cutting Boards: Scrub with a damp cloth and a handful of salt. Wood cutting boards will be brighter, cleaner and also smell fresher.

Wok: Cast-iron woks often rust when you wash them in water. Don't wash your wok like a dish or regular pan. Rather, while your wok is still hot, pour in a quarter cup of salt and scrub it with a stiff wire brush. Wipe clean and apply a light coating of sesame or vegetable oil before storing it away. Caution: Please do not use this approach on a non-stick surface, as it could scratch the coating!

Salt Secrets: Salt Tips for Life

You must salt every meal offering. Do not leave out the salt of your God's Covenant from your meal offerings.

- Leviticus 2:13

✱ Fifteen ✱

SALT TIPS FOR A SWEET HOME

As Nacell, our natural salt guru, explains, salt can sweeten your life and your home. Many people spray a natural salt mixture to bring the smell of the sea into their home. Is the occasional or frequent salt mist of benefit? Yes and no.

While the mister puts salt in the air, it all depends on how much salt you need. For instance, using several continuous "salt water mist dispensers" in a small room could potentially result in too much salt, but in a 4000 square foot home, you might to use want a few from time to time. Everything in moderation! A continuous salt mist could corrode silver and other precious items.

And please speak with your doctor to make sure that frequent or continuous salt mists are safe for your condition or conditions.

Salt Secrets: Salt Tips for Life

Salt Tips to Feng Shui Your Home

Feng Shui your home with natural salt. Place an assortment of salt crystals in any open area or passageway to energize the space. Sprinkle the salt around the perimeter of the room to absorb and clear negative energy. However, be sure to vacuum up and/or discard the salt within a day or two.

According to Feng Shui experts, strategic placement of energetic salt lamps, candleholders or crystals can also help attract abundance, wealth and love!

Salt Tips for Light Cleaning

Use natural salt for flowers and crafts, light cleaning, laundry and energy clearing. Stick with inexpensive or industrial salt for heavy grime, for snow removal and for dousing grease flames.

Artificial Flowers: Combine a tablespoon of salt with artificial flowers in a brown paper bag.

Salt Secrets: Salt Tips for Life

Shake a bit and remove the flowers. They'll sparkle.

Bottles and Containers: Remove the odor from bottles, pitchers and all containers. Salt can be used to clean and deodorize thermos bottles, plastic storage containers, pitchers and other closed containers. Pour a teaspoon of salt in the container, add a bit of water and let it sit for a few hours.

Drip-Proof Candles: Mix a half tablespoon of salt in two cups of water. Soak wax candles in the solution for two hours. The invisible crust that forms on the surface will encase future melted wax.

General Odors: Add a sweet smell by mixing some powdered cinnamon into the salt before using it.

Natural Air Freshener: No more expensive air fresheners! Just layer rose petals, lavender blossoms, orange peels, or other favorite fragrant blossoms with natural mineral salt in a pretty jar with a tight-fitting lid. Remove the lid to freshen

Salt Secrets: Salt Tips for Life

the room. You can renew the scent with a few drops of pure essential oil.

Natural Dehumidifiers. You can also use salt chips in your closets as natural dehumidifiers. I keep a very large Himalayan rock in a bowl in my front closet. When water accumulates, I simply pour it out. Unlike other mold or mildew prevention products, I never have to replace the rock! I simply wipe the rock with a towel.

Onions: Let garlic be your guide. Remove onion smells from your hands by rubbing your fingers with salt.

Salt Tips for Laundry

Iron: Use salt to can clean the surface of most irons (check with your manufacturer). Turn the iron on high. Sprinkle salt onto a piece of newspaper on your ironing board. Run the hot iron over the crystals to clean the surface.

Laundry Pre-treatment: Drown the spot in salt to absorb the grease. Wash as usual.

Salt Secrets: Salt Tips for Life

New Towels: Add one cup of salt to the wash. Salt will help set the colors so your towels remain bright much longer.

Perspiration Stains: Remove stubborn perspiration stains. Dissolve four tablespoons salt in one quart of hot water. Sponge the garment until the stain disappears.

Sneakers: Reduce odor and moisture by occasionally sprinkling a little salt in your canvas shoes.

Salt Tips for Stains and Drains

Bath Tub: Put a cup of salt into a gallon of filtered water. Let the salt dissolve and then pour it into a spray bottle. Shake the bottle and spray the enamel. Wipe it down with a cloth. Rinse the tub thoroughly.

Brass and Copper Polish: To shine candlesticks or remove green tarnish from brass or copper pots, make a paste of equal parts salt, flour, and vinegar. Rub with a soft cloth, then rinse with

Salt Secrets: Salt Tips for Life

warm, soapy water and buff back to its original shine.

Brooms: Soak your new bristle broom in a strong solution of hot salty water. Let it dry. Your broom will last much longer.

Copper Artwork: To remove stains and to freshen the patina, use a wash cloth or brush to gently rub salt into the copper. Rub the item a second time with a bit of vinegar.

Garbage Disposal: Toss a half cup of salt in your sink. Wipe the salt over the entire surface with a wet cloth. Then wash the salt down the drain and run the disposal to remove caked on materials and odors.

Hair-Clogged Drains: Combine one cup of salt, one cup baking soda and a half cup of white vinegar. Pour the mixture down the drain. After ten minutes, pour boiling water down the drain. Run hot water until the drain flows freely.

Oil or Grease on Carpet: Mix one part of salt to four parts of rubbing alcohol. Rub the solution

Salt Secrets: Salt Tips for Life

into stain in the direction of the nap of the rug. The oil or grease should rise to the surface. Vacuum the residue.

Red Wine Stains on Carpet: While the red wine is still wet, pour a bit of white wine on the stain to dilute the color. Dab the spot with a sponge and cold water. Sprinkle with salt, wait a few minutes and then vacuum the area.

Silver: Rub salt into tarnished silver with a wet cloth. The tarnish will wash off in the sink or dishwasher.

Vases: Remove flower stains by sprinkling salt on the bottle by hand or brush. Scrub the stain away.

Watermarks on Wood: Mixing one teaspoon of salt with a few drops of water to form a paste. Rub the paste onto the watermark with a soft cloth or sponge. Polish the wood.

Wicker: Scrub your wicker with salt water and a stiff brush to renew the natural color. Repeat this process as necessary.

Salt Secrets: Salt Tips for Life

Sponges: To make sponges like new again, soak them overnight in a solution of about 1/4 cup salt per quart of water.

Salt Tips for Home Fires & Ice

Barbecue Flame Retardant: Sprinkle salt on barbecue coals to reduce flames from meat drippings.

Fireplace: Douse your fireplace flames with salt to put them out safely.

Frost-free indoor windows and tracks: Rub the inside of windows with a sponge dipped in a saltwater solution. This will help prevent frost in sub-freezing weather. You can also sprinkle salt in the tracks so the window will open more easily. (Check with your window manufacture to determine if salt can be safely applied to their indoor windows.)

Grease Fires: If a grease fire should erupt, toss salt on the fire to extinguish the flames. *Never* pour water on a grease fire – the grease will splatter and spread the fire.

Salt Secrets: Salt Tips for Life

Salt Tips for Car and Driveway

Driveway: Salt is the primary element in costly industrial deicing products. Use inexpensive salt on your icy driveway to dry the ice and to smoothen the surface.

Windshield: Salt reduces the temperature at which water freezes. Wipe down your car windows and windshields with a sponge dipped in salt water and let them dry. During the winter, keep a small cloth bag of salt in your car. When the windshield and other windows are wet, rub with the salt bag to prevent ice formations. First, moisten the cloth bag filled with salt. Toss it about for a few minutes to create loose salt. Rub the cloth bag on your car's windshield to keep snow and ice from collecting.

Salt Tips for the Garden

Ants: Sprinkle Salt across your door frame or directly on the paths of ant trails. Ants will be discouraged from crossing this barrier.

Salt Secrets: Salt Tips for Life

Flowerpots: Sprinkle salt on soiled flowerpots. Scrub off the dry dirt with a stiff brush. It's easier and faster than water.

Poison Ivy: To help eliminate poison ivy, combine one ounce of soap and 24 ounces of salt in a gallon sprayer. Spray poison ivy leaves and stems with the solution.

Snails and Slugs: Pour a bit of salt or salty water on snails and slugs to eliminate them.

Unwelcome Plants: Bring a solution of two parts salt and one part water to a boil. Pour directly on unwelcome plants.

Salt Tips for Pets

All Pets: Harmonizes room energy for your pet! Pets are attracted to natural light and they sense the flow of energy within a room. Salt lamps and candleholders create positive room energy, while the rich array of colors can be especially calming for your pet. They also safeguard your pet by combating electro-smog, including computers, televisions and cell-phones.

✫ Sixteen ✫

YOUR HIDDEN SALT TREASURE

According to an ancient Chinese legend, you salt treasure is within reach if you seek the truth and have the patience to investigate.

China's phoenix, or feng-huang, is a beautiful bird with blue eyes and a scarlet head, breast and back. The feng-huang is also known as a noble and wise creature that hovers over treasures and bring fortune to those who see it.

One day a poor, hardworking peasant walked to his marshy fields long day's work. Suddenly he stopped and his eyes opened wide, for half-hidden among the reeds stood the fabulous feng-huang.

The peasant quickly ran toward the marsh, but as he reached the spot where the creature stood, it soared into the sky and disappeared. The peasant turned to the spot where the feng-huang had been

Salt Secrets: Salt Tips for Life

sitting. "There must be treasure buried here," he said and began to dig as fast as he could.

He dug and dug, but turned up only dirt and mud. At long last, he picked up a piece of earth and pondered. "This dirt must be the treasure," he said, and gazed up to the heavens. "The feng-huang promises treasure," he said softly. And so he wrapped the piece of earth in cloth and hurried home.

When he ran through the door, the peasant called to his wife, "I have found treasure," and he told her his tale. The two stared in wonder at the piece of earth.

"Dear husband," she said, "you know you must take this to the Emperor." The man nodded, for he knew, like everyone else in his country, that anyone who found a treasure must report it to the Emperor.

The peasant dressed in his work clothes, for these were the only clothes he owned. His wife carefully wrapped the piece of earth and placed it in a willow basket. Then the peasant took the basket in

Salt Secrets: Salt Tips for Life

his hands and walked all the way to the capital city. There he announced his wish to present a treasure to the Emperor .

When the Emperor asked to see the gift, the peasant bowed low, reached into his basket and held out the earth. He told the Emperor the tale of the magical phoenix. The Emperor frowned. "You are trying to make a fool of me, " he cried. "This is no treasure. Guards, take this man to the dungeon and put him to death. No one tries to trick the Emperor!"

The Emperor's guards obeyed their master. As for the basket of dirt, one of the servants placed it upon a shelf in the royal kitchen, and there everyone soon forgot all about it.

Some time later, one of the cooks was carrying a bowl of soup into the royal dining hall. As he walked, he passed beneath the basket, and a small clod of earth splashed into the soup. The cook was horrified, but just then the Emperor boomed, "Bring me my soup!"

Salt Secrets: Salt Tips for Life

The cook quickly carried the bowl to the table and placed it before the Emperor. His hands trembled and sweat poured from his brow as the Emperor dipped his spoon into the soup. The Emperor took one taste and smiled. "Delicious, " he said. this is the best soup I have ever tasted! What did you add to it?"

Still the cook trembled. "Your majesty," he began, "I did nothing special, but a bit of dirt from the peasant's basket fell into the soup. As he spoke, he turned as pale as the clouds.

The Emperor was amazed. "Bring me that basket," he called to his servants, for he remembered the peasant's tale of the feng-huang. When the basket sat before him, the Emperor reached in and sifted the earth through his hands. As he did, tiny white crystals clung to his palms.

"This is a treasure, " the Emperor said. "It is a gift from the phoenix. From this day on, we shall add these crystals to all of our dishes." He sent his men to dig in the earth where the peasant had first spied the phoenix. And that was how the people of China discovered salt and all its wonders.

Salt Secrets: Salt Tips for Life

The Emperor wept for the peasant he had punished with death. He sent for the man's wife and son. He placed the peasant's son in charge of all the lands where the white crystal gleamed in the soil.

The young man became rich and comfortable, and he cared well for his family. And so the peasant, honored through his son, rested in peace, and the feng-huang brought salt to China.*

* From "Tell Me a Story" – www.soupsong.com

Salt Secrets: Salt Tips for Life

The essence of salt is immutable. It can be evaporated back to its original crystalline shape even when dissolved in water.

Salt Secrets: Salt Tips for Life

✸ Seventeen ✸

SALT OVER GOLD

Salt is more valuable than gold when you have no salt. The following Czech fable beautifully illustrates the priceless value of salt.

Once upon time, there was a king who had three daughters. The king protected his daughters like the eyes in his head. When his limbs weakened and his head became white, he often thought about which of his three daughters should become the queen after his death. It was a difficult choice for him, because they all were shapely, and he loved each of them equally. At last it occurred to him to appoint the daughter who loved him most as the next queen.

He summoned his daughters and addressed them, "My daughters, as you can see, I am old, I do not know whether I will be with you much longer. Therefore, I want to appoint the one among you who will become the queen after my death. But before I do that, I would like to know how much

Salt Secrets: Salt Tips for Life

you love me. "Well now, my oldest daughter, tell me as the first, how much you love your father."

"My father, I love you more than gold!" his oldest daughter answered, and she kissed her father's hand.

"Well, now, my middle daughter, how much do you love your father?"

"Alas, my dear father, I love you like my green maiden wreath!" said the middle daughter, hugging her father around his neck.

"That is fine! What about you, my youngest daughter? How much do you love me?"

"Daddy, I love you like salt!" Maruška said as she looked at her father with a lovely smile.

"Eh, you, good for nothing, do you appreciate your father only as much as salt?" shouted her older sisters. "Of course, I love him as much as salt!" consented Maruška once more, and she looked at her father even more charmingly. But

Salt Secrets: Salt Tips for Life

she could not gain any understanding from her father either. Her father became immensely angry.

His youngest child appreciated her own father only as much as worthless salt – salt that is taken by everyone between their fingers and spilled.

"Go, go away from my eyes!" he shouted at her. "You don't value me more than you value salt! When the time comes that salt is worth more than gold, then you can become the queen."

Maruška could not say a word because of her sorrow. How could her father misjudge her love in such a way? She was used to obeying her father's orders without question and she knew that she would not be able to stay with her sisters in the house. She took her clothes and went away. She wandered through mountains and valleys aimlessly, and after some time, she came to a dark forest. An old woman stood in her way.

"Maruška, dear Maruška, tell me where you are going and why you are crying?"

Salt Secrets: Salt Tips for Life

"Ah, old lady, why should I talk to you? You can't help me?"

"Eh, my dear maiden. Just tell me about your problem. Perhaps, you can get a piece of advice from me. Don't you know that where there is gray hair, there is knowledge?"

Maruška told the old woman about her troubles. She just wanted to live to persuade her father that she loves him. The old woman knew what Maruška wanted to tell her because she was a clever woman, a prophetess. Therefore, she agreed with everything that Maruška told her and asked the young girl to serve her. Maruška was glad that she had found somebody to talk to about her troubles. With pleasure, she went with the old woman to her small cottage under the pines. The old woman offered Maruška what she had, and Maruška enjoyed the refreshments because she was both hungry and thirsty.

"And now," said the old woman, "you must go briskly to work. But do you know how to spin, spool and weave? Will you tend my flock of sheep, and will you milk them too?"

Salt Secrets: Salt Tips for Life

"I don't know how to do these things, but I will learn if you show me just once how to do it," said Maruška.

"Well, I'll show you everything, and when time finds its time, it will come in handy for you."

Maruška was very diligent, like a wasp into fruit, although she still did not know what it was like to live in a poor person's home. She soon became accustomed to everything. Rolled-up sleeves and a white apron suited her, just as if she were a capable maid.

During this time the other sisters lived very well. They spent time caressing their father, embracing him around his neck, pretending to show great love for him, because he gave them whatever they asked for.

Day by day, the oldest sister wore more and more expensive dresses and, day by day, adorned herself with gold. The middle sister organized feasts and dances. They were both satisfied, since they used their father's wealth as they wanted. The king soon noticed that his oldest daughter

Salt Secrets: Salt Tips for Life

loved gold more than her father. When the second daughter revealed to him that she would like to get married, he knew that her love would soon vanish also. The king thought about Maruška more than once, but what was he to do now? There was no news about her.

"Eh, what am I to do? She loved me as much as common salt," and he drove away his memory of her.

Once, there was to be a great feast at the castle. Perhaps the suitors were to visit the middle daughter. Suddenly, the cook came running breathlessly to the king. "My king," he stammered, "a great problem, there's a great problem!"

"What is happening with you? Have you lost your common sense?" asked the king.

"That is it, my king! My brain does not want to understand this! All the salt we had either became moist or disappeared as if it fell onto the ground. There is not a grain of salt anymore. How shall I salt the food now?"

Salt Secrets: Salt Tips for Life

"You, fool, have other salt brought to you!"

"Where can I get other salt? The same has happened in each house of your kingdom, and there is no salt in the entire country!"

"Well now! Prepare such meals for which salt is unnecessary!" said the nervous king. The cook thought to himself that it had to be, since the king ordered it so. At first, he cooked meals without salt, and then he cooked meals with what came to his mind, and at last, only sweet meals. Those were strange unsalted feasts. The guests left one after the other, and new guests did not come. Why should anyone come when he could not receive even what the poorest man has – bread, salt and good will. The king was annoyed! The daughters were stunned. Where was their golden time?

Of course, look! There was gold enough, but not a grain of salt, even though they sent messengers to the edge of the world. All the salt had disappeared. Gradually, people lost their inclination for living. Everybody wanted to have salt, just a little bit of salt on the tongue. Even the cattle suffered. Cows and sheep lost their milk

Salt Secrets: Salt Tips for Life

because they did not have any salt. People moved about stunned and sickly. The king and his daughters looked like shadows and could not be recognized because of their diseases. It was God's punishment for the whole country. The king proclaimed that whoever brought a grain of salt to him would be rewarded as much gold as his weight.

Now the king finally understood the true value of God´s salt. He would suffer his misery, but he had great pangs of conscience, because of Maruška and the injustice he had done to her. In the meantime, Maruška was very well. There was no work she could not learn or get used to. She knew nothing about misery, what had happened in her father's house or in her father's country. But the clever old woman knew about everything, and she also knew the right time would come for situations to be resolved. Therefore, she decided to talk to Maruška and she told her this: "My dear, I told you once that the right time would come when appropriate, even though much time might pass. Your time to return home has come."

Salt Secrets: Salt Tips for Life

"Oh, my dear granny, how can I go home when my father does not want me?" asked Maruška, as she burst into tears.

"Well, do not cry, my dear. Everything will be all right. Salt has become more expensive than gold in your country."

And then the old woman told Maruška everything that she had not known and added at the end, "You served me honestly, and, tell me now, what are you asking for your faithful service?"

"You advised me well, and you fed me well, granny. I thank you for everything. I'm asking for nothing special, just a handful of salt that I would like to bring as a present to my father."

"Do you not ask for anything else? Do you not know, that I can carry out everything?" asked the wise woman once more.

"I'm not asking for anything else, just for salt," answered Maruška.

Salt Secrets: Salt Tips for Life

"Well now! If you appreciate salt so much, never be lacking for it," said the prophetess for the last time. I will not give you anything more, just this switch. When you once feel a breeze blowing at noon, follow it. You will go through three valleys and over three mountains. Then stop and hit the ground with the switch! Where you hit the ground, it will open up and you will go inside. What you find there will be your dowry."

Maruška was grateful. She accepted the golden switch and a pouch of salt and left sadly, truly sadly. She was always in good standing with the old woman. She wanted to come to fetch her when she could arrange everything at home.

The old woman merely smiled and said, "My dear girl, remain as you are – good and honest – and you will live well forever. Do not worry about me in the least!" Speaking, they came to the edge of the forest. But when Maruška turned to thank the good old woman once more, she had disappeared. Maruška stood alone like a finger on her hand. She sighed after her father and hurried in the direction towards his castle.

Salt Secrets: Salt Tips for Life

She came to her home. Since she had not been seen for a long time, and since she wore a kerchief on her head, she was not recognized and was not allowed to go to the king. "Oh, just let me inside," insisted Maruška. "I´m bringing the king a special gift, more valuable than gold. Surely, he will become healthy from this medicine."

The king was told about this and ordered that the girl be brought to him at once. When Maruška entered the king's hall, she asked for bread. The king ordered bread to be brought to her, but sighed deeply, "We have bread but no salt!"

"What we did not have, that we can have now," said Maruška, who cut off a slice of bread, unfolded her little pouch with salt, sprinkled the bread with it and presented it to the king.

"Salt," rejoiced the king. "Well, my dear, that is a precious gift. How can I reward you? Ask for what you want. You will get everything that you ask for!"

"I´m not asking for anything, father, just love me as you love the salt!" Maruška said with a lovely

Salt Secrets: Salt Tips for Life

voice such as she used before and took away the kerchief from her head. The king nearly fainted with joy when he recognized his Maruška. He begged her not to complain about what had happened. She just embraced him and did not drop her eyes from him.

The news about the arrival of the king's youngest daughter extended at once from the castle to the town. The news quickly spread among the people that Maruška brought salt. Everyone was joyful. Maruška's sisters were also glad, not so much for their sister's return, as for the salt that she brought. They wanted to taste at least a little. Maruška forgot about the unfairness of her sisters and offered them a slice of bread with salt, too. Everybody who came to the castle received salt from her pouch. Her father admonished her that she should not give away all the salt, since it is said, "With the good only slowly."

Maruška simply answered, "There is still enough salt here, father." And really, she could take as much as she wanted, and there was still enough for everybody, as if salt would be in the pouch forever. Everyone recovered from their diseases as

Salt Secrets: Salt Tips for Life

if they had been in the sun! The king's disease disappeared, as if somebody took it away. Joyfully, he summoned the older advisors of the town and the whole country. Maruška was appointed the queen! At the very moment Maruška was proclaimed queen under the high heavens, she felt a pleasant warm breeze blowing into her face. It was noon. At once, she told her father everything that the clever old woman ordered her to do.

She followed the breeze, and after she went through three valleys and over three mountains, she stopped and whipped the ground with the switch. When she whipped the ground, an opening appeared, and Maruška went into the opening. Suddenly, she found herself in a large hall which was like ice. The ceiling, the walls, and the floor - everything sparkled and glimmered as if sparks were thrown about. There were glittering galleries at the sides from which small male dwarfs came running with burning lamps to welcome Maruška.

"Welcome, welcome, our queen. We have been waiting for you! Our mistress ordered us to show

Salt Secrets: Salt Tips for Life

you around everywhere and to show you everything, because everything here is yours." The dwarfs warbled, waved with their lamps and turned around her. They crept up and down the walls like flies. The walls glittered like jewels. Maruška walked as if blinded by this beauty. The dwarfs showed her around halls and galleries where icicles, hanging from the ceiling, glittered like silver. They led her into the garden where red icy roses, marigolds and other flowers, which were astonishing, could be seen.

The small men picked the nicest rose and handed it to their new queen. Maruška smelled it, but the rose had no a scent. "What is this?" asked the queen. "Indeed, I have never seen such beauty."

"All of this is salt," the dwarfs replied. Can salt really grow here Maruška wondered. She thought to herself that it would be a pity to take the least amount of it away. But the dwarfs guessed what she was thinking and called, "Take as much as you would like to. You will never take it all. You will never be lacking salt again!" Maruška thanked the small men politely, took leave of them and left the cave. But the cave stayed opened behind her.

Salt Secrets: Salt Tips for Life

When she returned home, she showed her father the rose and told him everything that had happened. The king saw that the old clever woman from the cottage gave his daughter a richer dowry than he could have ever given her. But Maruška did not forget the old woman from the poor cottage either. She had a beautiful carriage harnessed, and together with her father, she went to look for the old woman. She did not want to part from her.

Maruška knew the way to the cottage well because she knew each path in the forest. Even though they crossed the forest a hundred times, there was no sign of the cottage and its inhabitant. Now they were certain as to what kind of old woman she was. All of their searching would be futile, so they returned home. There was no salt in the given pouch any more, but Maruška knew where salt grew. They took the salt, as they needed it, and still they have not taken all of it. To this day, they have never been lacking for salt.

This tale was told to Czech fiction writer Božena Ne'mcova by a servant in a spa at Sliac, Slovakia.

Wishing you a sweet salt journey!

Dr. Joyce

www.DrJoyceStarr.com
www.SaltSecrets.com
Phone: 1-786-693-4223

Salt Secrets: Salt Tips for Life

INDEX*

Salt Secrets: Salt Tips for Life

F
Facial scrub, homemade salt 91
Feng Shui 54, 88, 108, 139
Food preparation 99, 100

H
Halite 14-5
Halochamber 83
Halotherapy 62, 83
Harmony 47, 49
Healing 40, 75, 92, 96-7, 140
Himalayan Primal Sea Crystal Energy Pendants 97, 140
Himalayan Salt 39, 40, 81, 91, 94, 99,

I
Inclusions 20-2, 31, 34, 36, 40, 57, 60, 77, 79, 93
Ionization 86

K
Katen, Gerald 87
King of Salt 14
Kosher Salt 99

L
Light frequencies 42, 43

M
Masks, salt 67
Mineral inclusions 30, 35-7, 40, 140
Mold 51-2, 57, 110
Molecules 15, 18

N
Natural Salt Oasis 9, 13-4, 17, 19, 72
Novotny, Naomi 77

O
Ocean Atlantic Sea Salt 79

Salt Secrets: Salt Tips for Life

P
Persian salt lamps   44
Polish salt lamps   44
Primal Sea   12, 17, 20, 49, 66, 97, 140
Primal Sea Salt Spa   66, 140

R
Rock salt   30, 31

S
Salt
   baths   66, 79
   beauty regimes   72
   brine solution   39, 78
   candleholders   41, 44, 46, 54, 72, 85, 87, 95
   caves   21-2, 39, 57, 61-2, 83
   chunks, edible Himalayan   77
   conductivity   26
   decor 87
   deficit   50
   exotic bath   87
   ions   54, 86
   lamps   41-2, 44, 46, 53-4, 72, 85-8, 95, 116
   pendants   97
   pipes   63
   premier artisan   91
Salt Conveyor   17, 19, 20-1, 23
Salt Conductor   25
Salt for Heal Spurs   82
Salt for Soft Tissue Injuries   81
SaltWorks
Sound of salt   63-4

T
Table salt   5, 14, 31, 38, 57, 65

[Created with **TExtract** / www.Texyz.com]

-141-

Salt Secrets: Salt Tips for Life

About the Author

Dr. Joyce Starr is an author, publisher and expert on natural healing. She established her niche publishing house in 2006. Dr. Joyce STARR Publishing specializes in books that Empower and Inspire. She has also authored books in diverse arenas, including: international policy, environmental policy, public policy and dynamic wellness strategies. Harper Collins, Henry Holt, Praeger, Contemporary Books and Westview Press published her works.

Her commentaries have appeared in leading newspapers – including the *Washington Post, Washington Times, Miami Herald, LA Times, International Herald Tribune* and *Jerusalem Post* – and numerous online media.

Dr. Starr has designed programs and centers of excellence for prominent think tanks and universities. She also organized three global water summits, serving as co-chair with the UN Secretary General and with heads of state. She consults with firms in cutting-edge arenas.

Salt Secrets: Salt Tips for Life

By the Author

Living Younger

Salt Secrets:
Salt Tips for Life

Himalayan Salt Crystals:
Your Dynamic Wellness Guide

Condo & Homeowner Defense

Defend Your Condo & Homeowner Rights!
What You Must Do When the Board
Turns Your Life Upside Down

Inspirational

Faxes to God:
Messages to the Western Wall of Jerusalem

International

Covenant Over Middle Eastern Waters: Key to World
Survival

Kissing Through Glass: The Invisible Shield
Between Americans and Israelis

US Policy on Water Resources in the Middle East

Salt Secrets: Salt Tips for Life

Made in the USA
Middletown, DE
10 January 2023

21797780R00089